I.V. Therapy

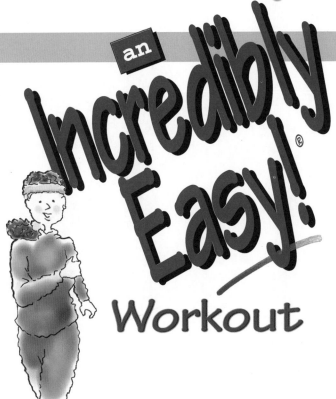

an **Incredibly Easy!** ®

Workout

I.V. Therapy

an Incredibly Easy!® Workout

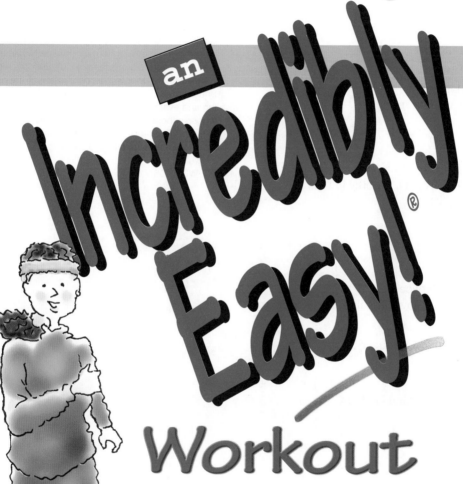

Wolters Kluwer | Lippincott Williams & Wilkins
Health

Philadelphia • Baltimore • New York • London
Buenos Aires • Hong Kong • Sydney • Tokyo

Staff

Executive Publisher
Judith A. Schilling McCann, RN, MSN

Editorial Director
David Moreau

Clinical Director
Joan M. Robinson, RN, MSN

Art Director
Mary Ludwicki

Editorial Project Manager
Gabrielle Mosquera

Clinical Project Manager
Jennifer Meyering, RN, BSN, MS, CCRN

Editor
Diane M. Labus

Copy Editors
Kimberly Bilotta (supervisor), Dorothy P. Terry

Designer
Lynn Foulk

Illustrator
Bot Roda

Digital Composition Services
Diane Paluba (manager), Joyce R. Biletz, Donald Knauss,
Donna S. Morris

Associate Manufacturing Manager
Beth J. Welsh

Editorial Assistants
Karen J. Kirk, Jeri O'Shea, Linda K. Ruhf

Workout regimen

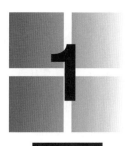

Fundamentals of I.V. therapy

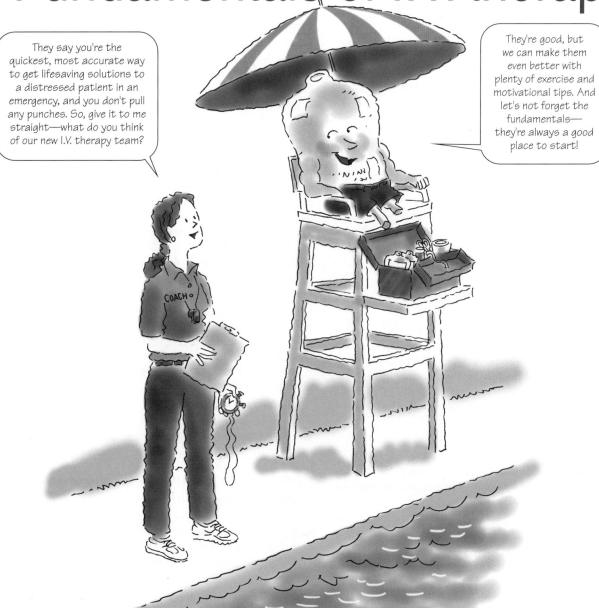

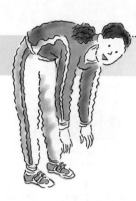

■■ **Warm-up**

Fundamentals of I.V. therapy review

Objectives of I.V. therapy

- To restore and maintain fluid and electrolyte balance
- To provide medications and chemotherapeutic agents
- To transfuse blood and blood products
- To deliver parenteral nutrients and nutritional supplements

Benefits

- Administers fluids, drugs, nutrients, and other solutions when a patient can't take oral substances
- Allows for more accurate dosing
- Allows medication to reach the bloodstream immediately

Risks

- Blood vessel damage
- Infiltration
- Infection
- Overdose
- Incompatibility of drugs and solutions when mixed
- Adverse or allergic reactions
- May limit patient activity
- Expensive

Fluids, electrolytes, and I.V. therapy

Fluid functions

- Helps regulate body temperature
- Transports nutrients and gases throughout the body
- Carries cellular waste products to excretion sites
- Includes intracellular fluid (ICF) (fluid existing inside cells) and extracellular fluid (ECF), which is composed of interstitial fluid (fluid that surrounds each cell of the body) and intravascular fluid (blood plasma)

Electrolyte functions

- Conducts current that's necessary for cell function
- Includes sodium and chloride (major extracellular electrolytes), potassium and phosphorus (major intracellular electrolytes), calcium, and magnesium

Fluid and electrolyte balance

- Fluid balance involves the kidneys, heart, liver, adrenal glands, pituitary glands, and nervous system.
- Fluid volume and concentration are regulated by the interaction of antidiuretic hormone (ADH) (regulates water retention) and aldosterone (retains sodium and water).

- The thirst mechanism helps regulate water volume.
- Fluid movement is influenced by membrane permeability and colloid osmotic and hydrostatic pressures.
- Water and solutes move across capillary walls by capillary filtration and reabsorption.

Types of I.V. solutions

Isotonic solutions

- Have the same osmolarity or tonicity as serum and other body fluids
- Include lactated Ringer's and normal saline
- Indicated for hypovolemia

Hypertonic solutions

- Have a higher osmolarity than serum and cause fluid to be pulled from the interstitial and intracellular compartments into the blood vessels
- Include dextrose 5% in half-normal saline and dextrose 5% in lactated Ringer's
- Used to reduce risk of edema, stabilize blood pressure, and regulate urine output

Hypotonic solutions

- Have a lower serum osmolarity and cause fluid to shift out of the blood vessels into the cells and interstitial spaces
- Include half-normal saline, 0.33% sodium chloride, and dextrose 2.5%
- Used when diuretic therapy dehydrates cells or for hyperglycemic conditions

I.V. delivery methods

- *Continuous infusion* provides constant therapeutic drug level, fluid therapy, or parenteral nutrition.
- *Intermittent infusion* administers drugs over a specified time.
- *Bolus injection* is used for a single-dose drug or solution.

Administration sets

- Selection depends on the type of infusion, infusion container, and need for volume-control device
- May be vented for those containers that have no venting system or unvented for those that do

Infusion flow rates

- Macrodrip delivers 10, 15, or 20 gtt/ml.
- Microdrip delivers 60 gtt/ml.

Calculating flow rates

- Divide the volume of the infusion (in ml) by the time of infusion (in minutes), and then multiply this value by the drop factor (in drops per ml).

Regulating flow rates

- Use clamps, volumetric pumps, or rate minders.
- Factors affecting flow rate include vein spasm, vein pressure changes, patient movement, manipulations of the clamp, bent or kinked tubing, I.V. fluid and viscosity, height of the infusion container, type of administration set, and size and position of the venous access device.

Checking flow rates

- Assess flow rates more frequently in patients who are critically ill, those with conditions that might be exacerbated by fluid overload, pediatric patients, elderly patients, and those receiving a drug that can cause tissue damage if infiltration occurs.

Professional and legal standards

- Events that may result in lawsuits include administration of the wrong dosage or solution, use of an incorrect route of administration, inappropriate placement of an I.V. line, and failure to monitor for such problems as adverse reactions, infiltration, and dislodgment of I.V. equipment.
- Professional and legal standards are defined by state nurse practice acts, federal regulations, and facility policy.
- To be eligible for reimbursement, compliance with standards of regulators is necessary.

Documentation of I.V therapy

When therapy is initiated, label the dressing on the catheter insertion site and the fluid container according to facility policy and procedures, and document:
- size, length, and type of device
- name of person inserting the device
- date and time
- site location
- type of solution and any additives used
- flow rate
- use of an electronic infusion device or other type of flow controller
- complications
- patient response
- nursing interventions

- patient teaching and evidence of patient understanding
- number of attempts.

Maintenance

Documentation for I.V. therapy maintenance includes:
- condition of the site
- site care provided
- dressing changes
- tubing and solution changes
- teaching and evidence of patient understanding.

Discontinued

Documentation for discontinuing I.V. therapy includes:
- time and date
- reason for discontinuing therapy
- assessment of site before and after venous access device is removed
- complications
- patient reactions
- nursing interventions
- integrity of the venous access device on removal
- follow-up actions.

Patient teaching

- Describe the procedure and why it's needed.
- State the solution to be infused and the estimated infusion time.
- Discuss activity restrictions.
- Consider using pamphlets, sample catheters, I.V. equipment, slides, or videotapes.
- Be honest about potential discomfort.
- Document the teaching and evaluate the patient's understanding.

■ Batter's box

Fill in the correct answers to these statements regarding I.V. therapy.

One of the most important nursing responsibilities is to administer _____ ,
1

_____ , and _____ to patients. In I.V. therapy,
2   3

_____ solutions are administered directly into the _____ ,
4   5

providing an immediate effect.

I.V. therapy is used to:

- restore and maintain fluid and _____ balance
  6

- provide medications and _____ agents
  7

- _____ blood and blood products
  8

- deliver parenteral nutrients and nutritional _____ .
  9

Options
A. chemotherapeutic
B. bloodstream
C. medications
D. supplements
E. fluids
F. electrolyte
G. liquid
H. blood products
I. transfuse

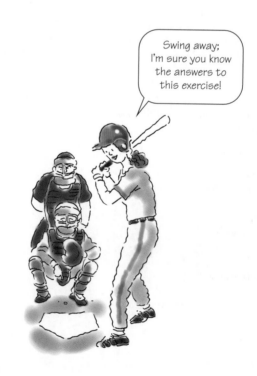

Swing away;
I'm sure you know
the answers to
this exercise!

Boxing match

I.V. therapy is an invasive procedure, and it doesn't come without risks. Using the syllables in the boxes and the clues provided, spell out the potential risks. The number of syllables for each answer is shown in parentheses. Use each syllable only once.

BIL	BLEED	COM	DOSE	FEC	~~FIL~~	I
I	IN	IN	~~IN~~	ING	O	PAT
~~TION~~	TION	~~TRA~~	TY	VER		

1. Infusion of I.V. solution into surrounding tissue rather than blood vessel

   (4) I N F I L T R A T I O N

2. Can occur with administration of too much I.V. solution or when response to drug is too rapid

   (3) __ __ __ __ __ __ __

3. May occur with mixing I.V. solution with another drug

   (7) __ __ __ __ __ __ __ __ __ __ __ __ __

4. Introduction of harmful microbes during administration of I.V. solution

   (3) __ __ __ __ __ __ __ __ __

5. Can occur when blood vessel is nicked, punctured, or otherwise damaged

   (2) __ __ __ __ __ __ __ __

> Whaddya say— are we in or out of this next exercise?

> Let's just go with the flow and hope for the best!

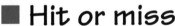

Hit or miss

Mark each statement with a "T" for "True" or an "F" for "False."

_____ 1. The human adult body is composed largely of liquid, accounting for about 80% of total body weight.

_____ 2. Body fluids are composed of water (a solvent) and dissolved substances (solutes).

_____ 3. Solutes in body fluids include electrolytes (such as sodium) and nonelectrolytes (such as proteins).

_____ 4. The two major body fluid compartments are ICF and intravascular fluid (also known as *plasma*).

_____ 5. The distribution of fluids between intracellular and extracellular body compartments normally fluctuates dramatically during the course of a day.

_____ 6. Interstitial fluid surrounds each cell of the body, even bone cells.

_____ 7. Most of the blood volume in the human body is made up of ICF.

_____ 8. The primary hormones responsible for regulating the body's fluid balance are ADH and aldosterone.

_____ 9. The thirst mechanism activates when water loss equals 10% or more of body weight or when osmolarity increases.

_____ 10. Drinking water restores plasma volume and dilutes ECF osmolarity.

Mind sprints

Go the distance by differentiating the signs and symptoms of fluid deficit and fluid excess you would expect to note during a patient assessment. Time yourself, and see how many findings you can list in 5 minutes.

Fluid deficit

- _____
- _____
- _____
- _____
- _____
- _____
- _____
- _____
- _____
- _____

- _____
- _____
- _____
- _____
- _____
- _____
- _____
- _____
- _____
- _____

> I'm just curious: Are we basing this exercise on standard time, daylight saving time, or the New York minute?

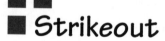

Fluid excess

- _____
- _____
- _____
- _____
- _____

- _____
- _____
- _____
- _____
- _____

Strikeout

Cross out the incorrect statements.

1. There are six major electrolytes found in body fluids: sodium, potassium, calcium, chloride, phosphorus, and magnesium.

2. Electrolyte imbalances rarely cause problems because the body can tolerate wide extremes in electrolyte levels.

3. All electrolytes dissociate in solution into electrically charged particles called *ions*.

4. Electrical charges of ions conduct current that's necessary for normal cell function.

5. Electrolytes are measured only in units of milliequivalents per liter (mEq/L).

6. A cation is an electrolyte with a negative charge.

7. The major intracellular electrolytes are potassium and phosphorus; the major extracellular electrolytes are sodium and chloride.

■ Match point

Match the electrolyte on the left with its principal functions and normal serum level on the right.

Electrolyte

1. Phosphorus _____
2. Calcium _____
3. Sodium _____
4. Chloride _____
5. Magnesium _____
6. Potassium _____

Principal functions and normal serum level

A. Major cation in ECF that influences water distribution; affects regulation of potassium, chloride, and acid-base balance; aids nerve and muscle fiber impulse transmission; normal serum level: 135 to 145 mEq/L

B. Major anion in ECF that helps maintain serum osmolarity and combines with other major cations to form important compounds; normal serum level: 96 to 106 mEq/L

C. Major cation in ICF that maintains cell electroneutrality and cell osmolarity; helps conduct nerve impulses, directly affects cardiac muscle contraction, and plays a major role in acid-base balance; normal serum level: 3.5 to 5 mEq/L

D. Major anion in ICF that helps maintain bone and teeth and cell integrity; acts as a urinary buffer in acid-base balance, promotes energy transfer to cells, and plays a major role in muscle, red blood cell, and neurologic function; normal serum level: 2.5 to 4.5 mg/dl

E. Cation in ICF that activates intracellular enzymes and carbohydrate and protein metabolism; acts on myoneural vasodilation and influences other cation movement; normal serum level: 1.5 to 2.5 mg/dl

F. Cation in ECF of teeth and bones that enhances bone strength and durability; helps maintain acid-base balance and affects activation, excitation, and contraction of cardiac and skeletal muscles; participates in neurotransmitter release, coagulation activation, and immune system function; normal serum level: 8.9 to 10.1 mg/dl

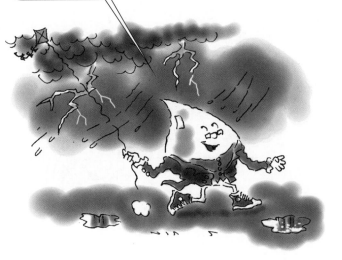

My latest experiment? Well, it has something to do with heat lightning, a large volume of water, and ionic charges.

Pep talk

"Diligence is the mother of good luck.
—Benjamin Franklin "

■ Power stretch

Stretch your knowledge of electrolytes a little further by unscrambling the words at left to reveal the name of five commonly encountered electrolyte imbalances. Then draw a line from the box to the signs and symptoms on the right.

> **Y C A M L H E C A P I O**
>
> — — — — — — — — — — — —

> **L A R M K Y E I P H E A**
>
> — — — — — — — — — — — —

> **H I M Y A T E A R O P N**
>
> — — — — — — — — — — — —

> **A N R E M P H Y I R A T E**
>
> — — — — — — — — — — — — —

> **P L A Y H I O K E M A**
>
> — — — — — — — — — — — —

A. Muscle weakness, muscle twitching, decreased skin turgor, headache, tremor, seizures, coma

B. Muscle tremor; muscle cramps; tetany; tonic-clonic seizures; paresthesia; bleeding; arrhythmias; hypotension; numbness or tingling in fingers, toes, and areas surrounding the mouth

C. Thirst; fever; flushed skin; oliguria; disorientation; dry, sticky membranes

D. Muscle weakness; nausea; diarrhea; oliguria; paresthesia of the face, tongue, hands, and feet

E. Decreased GI, skeletal muscle, and cardiac muscle function; decreased reflexes; rapid, weak, irregular pulse; muscle weakness or irritability; fatigue; decreased blood pressure; decreased bowel motility; paralytic ileus

---

Memory jogger

When working with fluids and electrolytes, remember that prefixes mean something and they always count!

Hypo- (as in "hypokalemia" or "hypotonic"): _____

Hyper- (as in "hypernatremia" or "hypertonic"): _____

Iso- (as in "isotonic"): _____

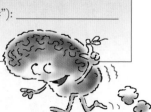

■ Batter's box

Not all electrolytes are distributed evenly in body fluid. Show you know the score by filling in the correct answers using the options given.

ICF and ECF contain different electrolytes because the _____

separating the two compartments have selective _____ , meaning

only certain ions can cross over. Although ICF and ECF have different solutes,

the _____ levels of the two fluids are about equal when balance is

maintained.

    The two ECF components— _____ and _____

(plasma)—have identical electrolyte compositions. The _____ in

capillary walls allow electrolytes to move freely between the two components,

allowing for equal distribution of electrolytes in both substances.

> **Options**
>
> A. interstitial fluid
>
> B. permeability
>
> C. concentration
>
> D. cell membranes
>
> E. intravascular fluid
>
> F. pores

According to my scorecard, it's the bottom of the eighth with three potassiums and four sodiums in the ICF, and two sodiums, two potassiums, and one magnesium in the ECF.

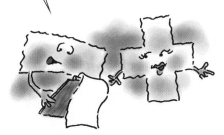

Pep talk

"The best and safest thing is to keep a balance in your life, acknowledge the great powers around us and in us. If you can do that, and live that way, you are really a wise man.
—Euripides"

■ Power stretch

Fluid movement is influenced by membrane permeability and colloid osmotic pressure. Unscramble the words on the left to reveal four common modes of moving solutes and fluid molecules through membranes. Then draw a line from each box on the left to its characteristics on the right. Note: Some characteristics may apply to two or more types.

A. Mode by which most solutes move

B. Mode in which molecules move by a physiologic pump mechanism, such as the sodium-potassium pump, to balance concentrations

C. Doesn't require energy; is considered a form of passive transport

SOSSIOM

— — — — — — —

D. Mode in which molecules move from an area of higher concentration to one of lower concentration

E. Forces fluid and solutes through capillary wall pores and into the interstitial fluid

IFUNFOIDS

— — — — — — — —

F. Mode in which movement between extracellular and intracellular compartments depends on osmolarity (concentration) of the compartments

AITECV   RTSATNPOR

— — — — — — —

— — — — — — — — —

G. Left unchecked, can cause plasma to move in one direction—out of the capillaries, causing severe hypovolemia and shock

H. Requires energy in the form of adenosine triphosphate for movement to occur

AAYCLLRPI   OIDUFINSF

— — — — — — — — —

— — — — — — — —

I. Mode in which molecules move from an area of lower concentration to one of higher concentration

J. Way in which fluids (particularly water) move

K. Mode in which substances move from area of higher hydrostatic pressure to one of lower hydrostatic pressure

■ You make the call

I know my being thin helps solutes pass through, but this is ridiculous!

Of all the vessels in the vascular system, only capillaries have walls thin enough to allow solutes to pass. Identify the related process illustrated here and describe what's happening in it.

Solutes

Capillary wall

Capillary

Hydrostatic pressure

Process: _____

_____

What's happening: _____

_____

_____

_____

_____

_____

Cross-training

Strengthen your knowledge of terms related to fluids and electrolytes by completing this crossword puzzle.

Across

3. Pressure at any level on water at rest due to the weight of water above it (two words)

6. Plasma fluid that makes up the liquid component of blood

7. Mechanism involving the passive movement of water

8. Major cation in extracellular fluid

10. Imbalance caused by a too-high chloride level

14. Solution having the same osmolarity as serum and other body fluids

15. Type of fluid found inside the cells, making up about 55% of total body fluid

Down

1. Energy-carrying molecule required for active transport (two words)

2. The concentration of a solution; is expressed in mOsm/L

4. Chemical compound that dissociates in solution into an ion

5. The only blood vessel with walls thin enough to allow solutes to pass through it

9. Transcellular fluid containing cerebrospinal fluid and lymph

11. Large protein found in capillary fluid

12. Most solutes move by this passive transport mechanism

13. Experienced when the body loses 2% of body weight or when osmolarity increases

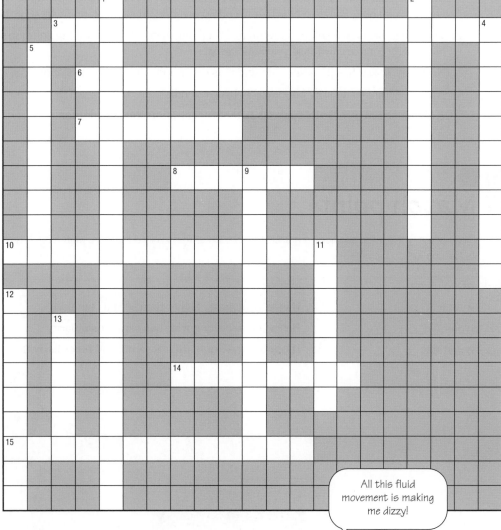

All this fluid movement is making me dizzy!

■ Hit or miss

Mark each statement with a "T" for "True" or an "F" for "False."

_____ 1. In any capillary, blood pressure normally exceeds colloid osmotic pressure up to the vessel's midpoint, and then falls below colloid osmotic pressure along the rest of the vessel.

_____ 2. The effect that an I.V. solution has on fluid compartments depends on the solution's osmolarity compared with serum osmolarity.

_____ 3. Normally, serum has the same osmolarity as other body fluids, which is about 150 mOsm/L.

_____ 4. A lower serum osmolarity may suggest hypovolemia.

_____ 5. A higher serum osmolarity suggests hemoconcentration and dehydration.

■ Match point

Three basic types of I.V. solutions are used to maintain or restore fluid balance. Match each type of solution on the left with its description on the right.

Type of solution

1. Isotonic _____

2. Hypotonic _____

3. Hypertonic _____

Description

A. Has an osmolarity higher than serum osmolarity

B. Has an osmolarity lower than serum osmolarity

C. Has the same osmolarity as serum and other body fluids

When it comes to fluids, maintaining and restoring balance is the name of the game.

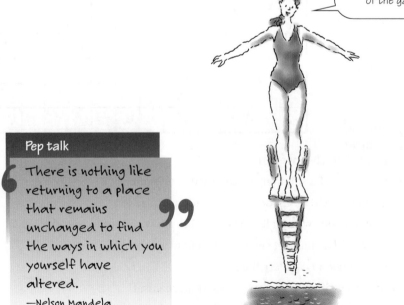

Pep talk

"There is nothing like returning to a place that remains unchanged to find the ways in which you yourself have altered."

—Nelson Mandela

You make the call

Identify the type of solution (isotonic, hypotonic, or hypertonic) pictured, and briefly explain how it changes or maintains body fluid status.

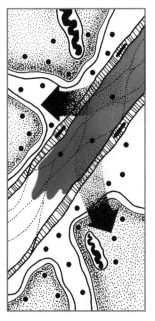

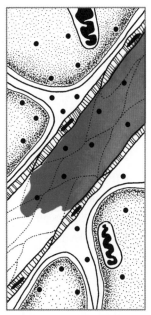

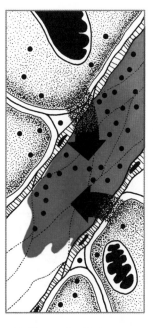

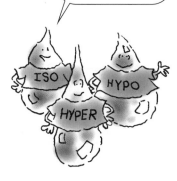

> Get moving! Once you pick up a pencil, the ideas should begin to flow.

1. Type of solution:

_____

2. Type of solution:

_____

3. Type of solution:

_____

How it changes/maintains body fluid status:

_____
_____
_____
_____
_____
_____
_____

How it changes/maintains body fluid status:

_____
_____
_____
_____
_____
_____
_____

How it changes/maintains body fluid status:

_____
_____
_____
_____
_____
_____

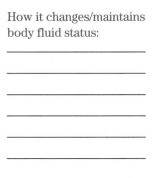

Pep talk

" The great pleasure in life is doing what people say you cannot do.
—Walter Bagehot "

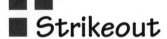

Team up!

Write each of the boxed solution names under the appropriate I.V. solution category. *Remember:* A solution is isotonic if it falls within (or near) the normal range for serum osmolarity. The osmolarity of each solution is provided.

Isotonic

_____

_____

_____

_____

_____

_____

_____

_____

Hypotonic

_____

_____

_____

_____

_____

Hypertonic

_____

_____

_____

_____

_____

_____

_____

_____

_____

Solutions
- 5% albumin (308 mOsm/L)
- 25% albumin (1,500 mOsm/L)
- Dextrose 2.5% in water (126 mOsm/L)
- Dextrose 5% in half-normal saline (406 mOsm/L)
- Dextrose 5% in lactated Ringer's (575 mOsm/L)
- Dextrose 5% in normal saline (560 mOsm/L)
- Dextrose 5% in water (260 mOsm/L)
- Half-normal saline (154 mOsm/L)
- Hetastarch (310 mOsm/L)
- Lactated Ringer's (275 mOsm/L)
- Normal saline (308 mOsm/L)
- Normosol (295 mOsm/L)
- Ringer's (275 mOsm/L)
- 0.33% sodium chloride (103 mOsm/L)
- 3% sodium chloride (1,025 mOsm/L)
- 7.5% sodium chloride (2,400 mOsm/L)

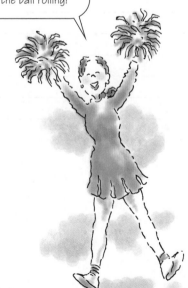

Gimmie an "I!" Gimmie a "V!" Hey, somebody's got to get the ball rolling!

Strikeout

Hypertonic solutions are commonly ordered postoperatively because the shift of fluid into the blood vessels offers several beneficial effects. Of the following effects, cross out the ones that aren't applicable to hypertonic solutions.

1. Regulate urine output

2. Stabilize blood pressure

3. Reduce fluid in the circulation

4. Reduce the risk of edema

5. Hydrate the cells

6. Increase intracranial pressure (ICP)

Batter's box

Some I.V. solutions can cause dangerous fluid shifts in patients with certain underlying conditions; therefore, their use may be contraindicated. Fill in the blanks with the correct answers using the options given.

- Lactated Ringer's is contraindicated if the patient's pH is greater than 7.5 because the liver converts _____ to _____ .

  $\underline{}_1$ $\underline{}_2$

- Hypotonic solutions are contraindicated in patients at risk for third-space fluid shifts, such as those with _____ , trauma, or low

  $\underline{}_3$

  serum _____ levels from malnutrition or liver disease.

  $\underline{}_4$

- Patients with impaired heart or kidney function shouldn't receive hypertonic solutions because of possible _____ .

  $\underline{}_5$

- Dextrose 5% in water is contraindicated for patients with increased _____ because it acts like a hypotonic solution, shifting

  $\underline{}_6$

  more fluid into cells and _____ .

  $\underline{}_7$

- Hypertonic solutions shouldn't be given to patients with conditions that can cause cellular dehydration such as _____ .

  $\underline{}_8$

- Patients who are at risk for increased ICP from _____ ,

  $\underline{}_9$

  head trauma, or _____ shouldn't receive hypotonic

  $\underline{}_{10}$

  solutions.

Options

A. bicarbonate

B. burns

C. diabetic ketoacidosis

D. fluid overload

E. ICP

F. interstitial compartments

G. lactate

H. neurosurgery

I. protein

J. stroke

After a hard workout, a relaxing soak in a whirlpool bath may be just the "tonic" you need.

Jumble gym

The I.V. route provides a rapid, effective way of administering various medications. Unscramble the names of the commonly infused drug classes listed below, and then use the scrambled letters to answer the question posed.

Question: Drugs may be delivered intravenously by bolus injection, by continuous infusion, or by what other type of infusion?

1. R A D I O R S L U C A V C A   S G R U D

 _ _ _ _ ◯ _ _ _ _ _ _ _ _   _ _ _ _

2. C O B S T I N A I T I   _ ◯◯ _ _ _ _ _ _ _

3. H O L Y M I T T S R O B C   _ _ _ ◯ _ _ _ _ ◯ _ _ _

4. I T H E A N M I S - R E T P E R O C   S A A T S G T O N N I

 _ _ _ _ _ _ _ _ _ ◯ - _ ◯ _ _ _ _ _ ◯   _ _ _ _ _ _ _ _ _ _ _

5. A L C S P T I E N I T A O N S   _ ◯ _ _ _ _ _ _ _ _ _ _ ◯ _ _

6. S C A N T V O S A T N I L U N   _ _ ◯ _ _ _ _ _ _ _ _ _ _ ◯ _

Answer: _ _ _ _ _ _ _ _ _ _ _

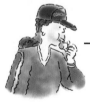

Coaching session

Are you able to label—correctly?

To label a dressing

To label a new dressing over an I.V. site, include:
- date of insertion
- gauge and length of venipuncture device
- date and time of dressing change
- your initials.

To label an I.V. bag

To label an I.V. solution container, include (in addition to the time tape):
- patient's name, identification number, and room number
- date and time the container was hung
- additives and their amounts
- flow rate
- sequential container number
- expiration date and time of infusion
- your name.

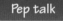

Pep talk

Determine never to be idle. It is wonderful how much may be done if we are always doing.

—Thomas Jefferson

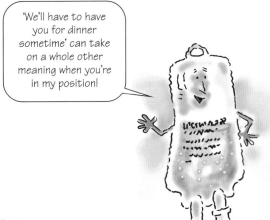

'We'll have to have you for dinner sometime' can take on a whole other meaning when you're in my position!

Mind sprints

Total parenteral nutrition (TPN) is a type of I.V. fluid that's customized for each patient. It includes a mixture of seven basic ingredients to meet the patient's energy needs and requirements. See if you can list all of the ingredients in 1 minute or less.

- _____
- _____
- _____
- _____
- _____
- _____
- _____

Strikeout

Cross out the incorrect statements.

1. TPN should be used only when the gut is unable to absorb nutrients.

2. A patient can receive TPN only up to 6 months.

3. TPN can cause liver damage if given long-term.

4. Peripheral parenteral nutrition (PPN) can be given indefinitely.

5. PPN is delivered by peripheral veins.

6. PPN solutions contain a lower amino acid concentration than TPN solutions.

7. Complications of PPN therapy include vein damage and infiltration.

8. Because TPN doesn't contain sugar, it isn't necessary to check the patient's glucose levels.

9. It's important to assess the patient's pancreatic enzymes (lipase, amylase trypsin, and chemotrypsin), triglycerides, and albumin levels when giving parenteral nutrition.

■ Batter's box

There are three basic methods for delivering I.V. therapy. Fill in the blanks below to complete the statements describing them. Use each option only once.

A _____ allows you to give a carefully regulated
      1

amount of fluid over a _____ period. With
               2

_____ infusions, a solution (commonly a medication
    3

such as an _____) is given for shorter periods at set
         4

intervals. With _____ (sometimes called *I.V. push*),
       5

a single dose of a drug is given.

> **Options**
> A. antibiotic
> B. bolus injection
> C. continuous infusion
> D. intermittent
> E. prolonged

■ Train your brain

Sound out each group of pictures or symbols to discover information about one type of I.V. infusion.

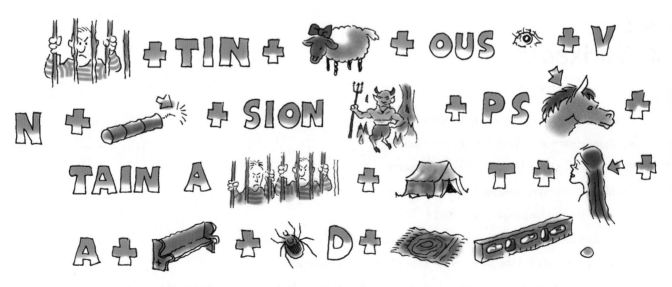

Finish line

Various veins can be used in peripheral and central venous therapy. Identify the veins pictured below.

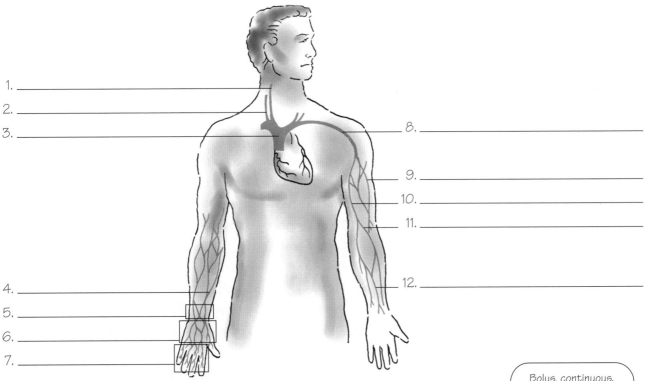

1. _____
2. _____
3. _____

4. _____
5. _____
6. _____
7. _____

8. _____

9. _____
10. _____
11. _____

12. _____

Match point

I.V. delivery methods have various uses. Match the type of I.V. delivery method on the left with the indication or use on the right. Note: Each indication or use may be used more than once.

I.V. delivery method

1. Intermittent infusion _____
2. Bolus injection _____
3. Continuous infusion _____

Indication or use

A. Consistent fluid levels are needed.

B. Drugs are needed for short periods, over varying intervals.

C. Patient requires an immediate high blood level of a medication.

D. A drug must be given quickly for an immediate effect in an emergency.

E. Steady, uninterrupted serum levels are needed.

F. Constant venous access is required but not a continuous infusion.

G. Two or more compatible admixtures must be administered continuously but at different rates.

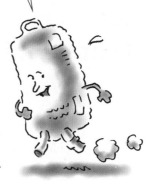

Bolus, continuous, intermittent—no matter how, we I.V.s always deliver!

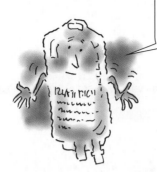

Who knew there were so many advantages to using intermittent infusions?

Power stretch

Stretch your knowledge of the benefits of intermittent infusion by first unscrambling the words at left to reveal common infusion delivery methods. Then draw a line from the box to its advantages at right.

ESANIL COKL

— — — — — —   — — — —

PIKBCYAGG HDTEMO

— — — — — — — — —

— — — — — —

EVMUOL– ORTOLCN EST

— — — — — — -

— — — — — — —   — — —

A. Requires only one large container

B. Avoids multiple I.M. injections

C. Provides high drug levels for short periods

D. Provides venous access for patients with fluid restrictions

E. Lowers cost

F. Prevents fluid overload from runaway infusion

G. Permits repeated administration of drugs through a single I.V. line

H. Preserves veins by reducing frequent venipunctures

I. Allows better patient mobility between doses

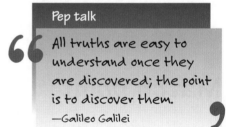

Pep talk

" All truths are easy to understand once they are discovered; the point is to discover them.
—Galileo Galilei "

Hit or miss

Some of the following statements about I.V. administration sets are true and others are false. Mark each statement with a "T" for "True" and an "F" for "False."

_____ 1. The choice of administration set largely depends on the type of infusion to be provided, the infusion container, and whether a volume-control device is needed.

_____ 2. I.V. administration sets come in three basic forms: vented, unvented, and circumvented.

_____ 3. Vented sets are used when containers have no venting system (such as for I.V. plastic bags and certain bottles).

_____ 4. I.V. administration sets are often equipped with ports for infusing secondary medications and filters for blocking microbes, irritants, and large particles.

_____ 5. The I.V. tubing packaged with administration sets is standardized because the same type is used for all patients.

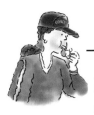

Coaching session

I.V. orders: Are they complete?

A complete order for I.V. therapy should always specify the following:
- type and amount of solution
- any additives and their concentrations (such as 10 mEq potassium chloride in 500 ml dextrose 5% in water)
- rate and volume of infusion
- duration of infusion.

Orders may be standardized for different illnesses and therapies, or they may be individualized. Some facilities dictate an automatic stop order for I.V. fluids (in many cases, 24 hours from the time they're written) unless otherwise specified. If an I.V. order is incomplete or seems inappropriate given the patient's condition, consult the practitioner.

Finish line

There are two basic types of flow rates available with I.V. administration sets: macrodrip and microdrip. Regardless of which set you use, the formula for calculating flow rates is the same. Fill in the missing formula information below.

1. Drops delivered by macrodrip (amount): _____

2. Drops delivered by microdrip (amount): _____

3. Formula for calculating flow rate: _____

4. How to adjust the flow to the calculated rate: _____

_____

_____

_____

Is anybody timing me? I think I may have just set a new flow rate world record!

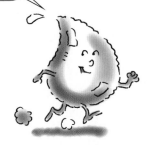

■■
■ Strikeout

A key aspect of administering I.V. therapy is maintaining accurate flow rates for solutions. Cross out the incorrect *word or phrase* in these statements.

1. Examples of commonly used infusion control devices include clamps, volumetric pumps, time tapes, water seal chambers, and rate minders.

2. Factors that can affect the flow rate include the type of I.V. fluid, the viscosity of the I.V. fluid, the height of the infusion container, the type of administration set, the size and position of the venous access device and the number of venipuncture attempts.

3. Factors that can affect the flow rate when using a clamp include number of hours of sleep, vein spasms, vein pressure changes, patient movement, manipulation of the clamp, and bent or kinked tubing.

4. Many nurses routinely check the flow rate whenever they're in a patient's room, every 15 minutes, and after each position change.

5. More frequent flow rate checks are required for patients who are critically ill, who have conditions that might be exacerbated by fluid overload, who complain of being cold, who are very young or elderly, or who are receiving drugs that can cause tissue damage if infiltration occurs.

■■
■ Jumble gym

Unscramble the following words to discover potential complications associated with infusion rates that are too fast or too slow. Then use the circled letters to answer the question posed.

Question: Secondary complications that can result from having too much fluid in the system include pulmonary edema and what other condition?

1. B E S T P I L I H _ ◯ _ _ _ _ _ ◯ _

2. F L A T I R O N I N T I _ _ ◯ _ _ _ _ ◯ _ _ _ _

3. T I Y O C A L U C R R   R V O L D A E O
   _ _ _ _ ◯ _ ◯ _ _ _ _   _ _ ◯ _ ◯ _ _ _

4. E E S R A V D   G U R D   A N R O C I T S
   _ _ _ ◯ ◯ _ _   _ _ _ _   _ ◯ _ _ ◯ _ _ _

Answer: _ _ _ _ _   _ _ _ _ _ _ _

■■
■ Mind sprints

Proper documentation of I.V. therapy is essential to nursing practice. In 2 minutes or less, list six different types of forms or documents on which I.V. therapy may be recorded.

- _____
- _____
- _____
- _____
- _____
- _____

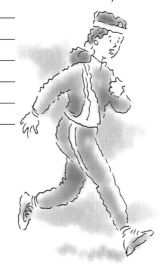

Don't give up now! Just a few more laps and we'll move on to the next chapter!

■■
■ Strikeout

When documenting the insertion of a venous access device or the beginning of therapy, you'll need to record several pieces of information. Cross out the items that *aren't* necessary to record.

1. Size, length, and type of the device

2. Name of the person who inserted the device

3. Date and time

4. Site location (anatomical name preferred)

5. Time of patient's last meal and bowel movement

6. Type of solution

7. Solution's manufacturer and expiration date

8. Any additives

9. List of potential interactions

10. Flow rate

11. Use of an electronic infusion device or other type of flow controller

12. Complications, patient response, and nursing interventions

13. Patient teaching and evidence of patient understanding

14. Number of attempts (both successful and unsuccessful)

■ Hit or miss

Mark each statement about documenting I.V. therapy with a "T" for "True" or an "F" for "False."

_____ 1. When documenting I.V. maintenance, specify the condition of the site, site care provided, dressing changes, tubing and solution changes, and your teaching and evidence of patient understanding.

_____ 2. When using an intake-output sheet for a child or a critically ill patient, you should record intake of all I.V. infusions (including fluids, medications, flush solutions, blood and blood products, and other infusates) every 3 to 4 hours.

_____ 3. Sequential numbering of all I.V. solutions administered to a patient can help reduce medication administration errors.

_____ 4. Recording the reason for discontinuing I.V. therapy isn't usually necessary unless the patient has complications.

_____ 5. Hourly output recorded on an intake-output sheet includes urine, stool, vomitus, gastric drainage, and any unused I.V. solution.

■ Jumble gym

Teaching about I.V. therapy includes preparing the patient for what to expect. Use the clues below to unscramble the four general areas on which to focus your teaching and the two common reactions your patient is likely to experience upon initiation of therapy. Then use the circled letters to answer the last question.

Not sure how I got the job, but I'm the official record keeper for all these exercises!

Question: Use of which techniques can help ease the patient's fears about I.V. therapy?

1. Should cover what, when, where, how, and why

E R P U D E C O R   _ _ _ _ _ _ ◯◯ _

2. For a child, can make this a show-and-tell experience

N I P M U T E E Q   ◯_ _ _ _ _ ◯_ _

3. Usually doesn't last too long   M I D C O F R O S T   ◯_ _ _ ◯_ _ _ _ _

4. Can put a kink in your patient's plans or a crimp in his style

T C A Y V I T I   R N O S C T R S I T E I
_ ◯_ _ _ _ _ _   ◯_ ◯_ _ _ _ _ _ _ ◯_

5. May be felt as the needle goes in

N R E S T T A I N   P I N A   ◯_ _ _ _ _ _ _ ◯   _ _ _ ◯

6. Can feel shocking at first   O L C D   E S T A I N S O N
_ _ _ _   ◯_ _ _ _ ◯_ _

Answer: _ _ _ _ _   _ _ _ _ _ _ _ _ _

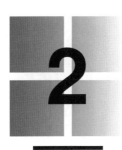

Peripheral I.V. therapy

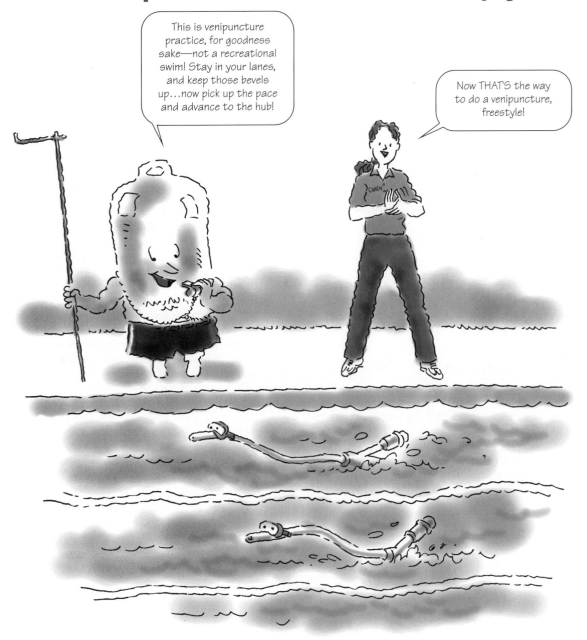

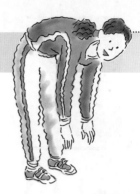

Peripheral I.V. therapy review

Basics of peripheral I.V. therapy

Peripheral I.V therapy involves:
- checking the practitioner's orders
- ordering supplies and equipment
- labeling solutions and tubing
- documenting nursing interventions.

Peripheral I.V. therapy is ordered when venous access is needed for:
- surgery
- transfusions
- emergency care
- maintaining hydration
- restoring fluid and electrolyte balance
- providing fluids for resuscitation
- administering I.V. medications or nutrients.

Preparing for venipuncture and infusion

- Review the practitioner's orders.
- Describe the procedure to the patient and provide patient teaching.
- Position the patient comfortably.
- Select the appropriate insertion site, venous access device, solution container, and administration set according to the therapy required. Then obtain an infusion pump.
- Label the container correctly and attach the administration set as appropriate.

Performing a venipuncture

- Dilate the vein, apply a tourniquet as appropriate, and prepare the access site.
- Stabilize the vein, and then position the venous access device with the bevel side up.
- Insert the device using a smooth, steady motion.
- Secure the venous access device.
- Document the procedure in the appropriate areas according to your facility's policy.

Maintaining peripheral I.V. therapy

- Focus on preventing complications.
- Discontinue the infusion when therapy is completed.
- Change a gauze dressing every 48 hours.
- Change the I.V. solution container when due or every 24 hours.
- Change administration sets every 72 hours.
- Change the I.V. site every 48 to 72 hours according to facility policy.
- Document dressing, tubing, and solution changes, and the condition of the venipuncture site.

Patients with special needs

- Infant I.V. sites include the dorsum of hand, feet, antecubital fossa, and scalp. Scalp veins are used for infants ages 6 months and younger.
- Intraosseous access is used for fluid resuscitation, medication administration, and blood transfusions until a vein can be accessed.
- Veins in elderly patients are more fragile and less elastic.

Complications of therapy

- Complications include infiltration, phlebitis, cellulitis, catheter dislodgment, occlusion, vein irritation or pain at the I.V. site, severed or fractured catheter, hematoma, venous spasm, vasovagal reaction, thrombosis, thrombophlebitis, and damage to the nerves, tendons, or ligaments, air embolism, allergic reactions, and septicemia.

■ ■ ■ Mind sprints

Peripheral I.V. therapy is ordered whenever venous access is needed. Time yourself and see how many common uses of I.V. therapy you can list in 1 minute.

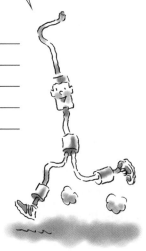

If I'm not mistaken, the peripheral route should be just up ahead, around the next bend.

■ _____
■ _____
■ _____
■ _____
■ _____

■ ■ ■ Strikeout

Few nursing responsibilities require more time, knowledge, and skill than administering peripheral I.V. therapy. Cross out the responsibilities that *don't* typically apply to this procedure.

1. Assembling equipment
2. Preparing the patient
3. Inserting a venous access device
4. Depositing all used catheters and needles in a double-bagged trash bin in the patient's bathroom
5. Regulating the I.V. flow rate
6. Monitoring for adverse effects
7. Checking the practitioner's orders and modifying them when necessary
8. Ordering and preparing supplies and equipment
9. Labeling solutions and containers
10. Teaching venipuncture to the nurse's aide
11. Documenting nursing interventions
12. Discontinuing all I.V. solutions at the end of shift

Pep talk

❝ It is confidence in our bodies, minds, and spirits that allows us to keep looking for new adventures, new directions to grow in, and new lessons to learn—which is what life is all about. ❞

—Oprah Winfrey

■ Strikeout

Cross out all of the items you *don't* need to check for on a patient's medical record before a venipuncture.

1. Allergies
2. Height
3. Disease history
4. Current diagnosis
5. Family history
6. Last medication given
7. Doctor's orders
8. Lab reports
9. Last hospitalization

■ Boxing match

Peripheral I.V. therapy is an invasive vascular procedure that carries some risks. To find out some of the associated risks, fill in the answers to the clues below by using all the syllables in the boxes. The number of syllables for each answer is shown in parentheses. Use each syllable only once.

~~AGE~~	AGE	BLEED	~~DAM~~	DAM	FEC	FIL
HEAR	HEART	IN	IN	ING	ING	~~KID~~
LOSS	~~NEY~~	TION	TION	TRA		

1. May be detected by increased creatinine and blood urea nitrogen levels

    (4) <u>K I D N E Y</u> <u>D A M A G E</u>

2. Occurs when drugs or caustic substances enter tissue surrounding the vein

    (4) _ _ _ _ _ _ _ _ _ _ _

3. Sensory problem that can occur with rapid infusion of some drugs

    (3) _ _ _ _ _ _ _ _ _ _ _

4. Can occur with rough handling or a nicked vein

    (2) _ _ _ _ _ _ _ _

5. May occur with introduction of microorganisms

    (3) _ _ _ _ _ _ _ _ _

6. May result from fluid overload or rapid infusion of certain drugs

    (3) _ _ _ _ _ _ _ _ _ _ _ _

■ Hit or miss

Mark each statement about I.V. equipment with a "T" for "True" or an "F" for "False."

_____ 1. Besides the venous access device, peripheral I.V. therapy requires a solution container, an administration set, and possibly an in-line filter.

_____ 2. Most facilities use glass I.V. solution containers for routine administration of I.V. fluids.

_____ 3. Plastic solution containers reduce the risk of air embolism or airborne contamination because they collapse as fluid flows out and they don't require venting.

_____ 4. Vented I.V. administration sets have an extra filtered port near the spike that allows air to enter and displace fluid.

_____ 5. There are three major types of I.V. administration sets: basic, or primary; add-a-line, or secondary line; and volume-control.

_____ 6. In-line filters, located in a segment of the I.V. tubing, prevent large particles from entering the vein; however, they can't prevent smaller particles or air from passing through.

_____ 7. Selecting the correct administration set requires knowing the type of solution container and comparing the set's flow rate with the nature of the I.V. solution.

_____ 8. A more viscous solution requires the use of a microdrip system to deliver fewer drops per milliliter.

_____ 9. Depending on the type of therapy ordered, additional equipment (including stopcocks, extension loops, and needleless systems) may be needed.

_____ 10. Basic I.V. administration sets range from 70″ to 110″ (178 to 279 cm) long.

_____ 11. Add-a-line sets contain a backcheck valve to prevent backward flow of a secondary solution into the primary solution.

_____ 12. Volume-control sets deliver large quantities of fluid and therefore shouldn't be used with pediatric patients.

_____ 13. In-line filters range in size from 0.2 micron (most common) to 170 microns.

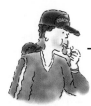

Coaching session
Using an in-line filter

Here are some general guidelines for using an in-line filter.
• When using a filter with an infusion pump, make sure it can withstand the pump's pressure. Some filters are made for gravity flow and may crack if the pressure exceeds a certain level.
• Make sure the filter is distal in the tubing and located close to the patient.
• Carefully prime the filter to eliminate all of the air from it.
• Change the filter according to the manufacturer's recommendations to prevent bacteria from accumulating and releasing endotoxins and pyrogens small enough to pass through the filter into the bloodstream.

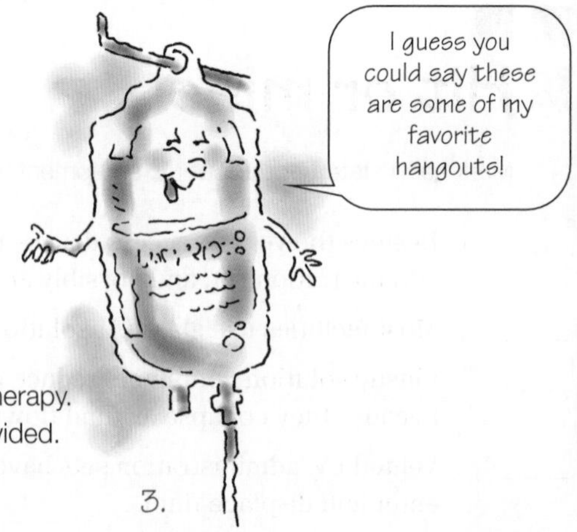

I guess you could say these are some of my favorite hangouts!

■■
■ You make the call

Three major types of I.V. administration sets can be used for peripheral I.V. therapy. Identify the sets shown here, and briefly explain their uses in the spaces provided.

1.

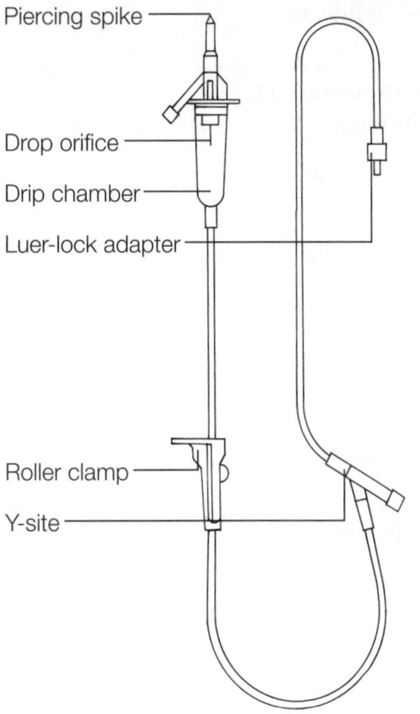

Piercing spike

Drop orifice

Drip chamber

Luer-lock adapter

Roller clamp

Y-site

2.

Piercing spike

Drop orifice

Drip chamber

Backcheck valve

Luer-lock adapter

Y-site

Y-site

Roller clamp

3.

Piercing spike

Roller clamp

Y-site

Volume-control chamber

Drop orifice

Drip chamber

Needleless adapter

Type of set: _____

_____

Uses: _____

_____

_____

_____

_____

_____

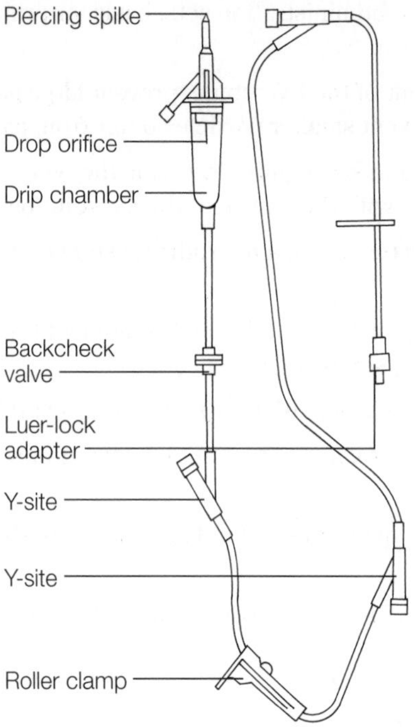

Type of set: _____

_____

Uses: _____

_____

_____

_____

_____

_____

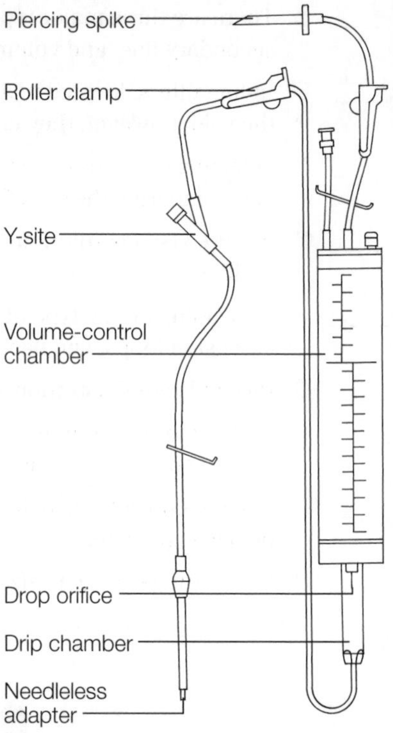

Type of set: _____

_____

Uses: _____

_____

_____

_____

_____

_____

■ Batter's box

Step up to the plate and take a swing at completing the missing information below. Use each answer option only once.

Because of their increased cost, in-line filters aren't routinely used. However, you can expect to use them in the following situations:

■ when treating an _____ patient
  ₁

■ when administering _____
  ₂

■ when using _____ composed of
  ₃

  many separate particles (such as

  _____ that require reconstitution)
  ₄

■ when the risk of _____ is high.
  ₅

> Options
>
> A. additives
>
> B. antibiotics
>
> C. immunosuppressed
>
> D. phlebitis
>
> E. total parenteral nutrition

■ Mind sprints

In 1 minute or less, list five reasons why you might discard an I.V. solution upon inspecting the solution container and its contents.

■ _____

■ _____

■ _____

■ _____

■ _____

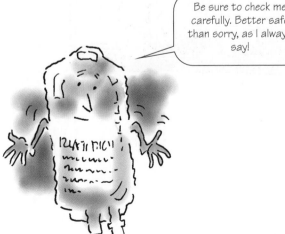

Be sure to check me carefully. Better safe than sorry, as I always say!

■ Match point

After the solution bag or container is attached, it's time to prime the administration set. Match the step on the right with the type of administration set on the left.

Type of administration set

1. Basic set _____
2. Add-a-line set _____
3. Volume-control set _____

Steps

A. Close the roller clamp below the drip chamber and squeeze the chamber until it's half full. Aim the distal end of tubing at a receptacle. Open the roller clamp and allow solution to flow through the tubing to remove air. Close the clamp after solution has run through the line and all air has been purged from the system. As solution flows back through the tubing, invert the backcheck valves so that solution can flow into them, tapping the valves to release any trapped air bubbles. Straighten the tubing and continue purging air in the usual manner.

B. Close the roller clamp below the drip chamber and squeeze the chamber until it's half full. Aim the distal end of the tubing at a receptacle. Open the roller clamp and allow solution to flow through the tubing to remove air. Close the clamp after solution has run through the line and all air has been purged from the system.

C. Attach the set to the solution container and close the lower clamp on the I.V. tubing below the drip chamber. Open the clamp between the solution container and the fluid chamber, allowing about 50 ml of solution to flow back into the chamber. Close the upper clamp, then open the lower clamp, allowing solution in the chamber to flow through the remainder of tubing. Make sure some fluid remains in the chamber so that air won't fill the tubing below it. Close the lower clamp. Fill the chamber with the desired amount of solution.

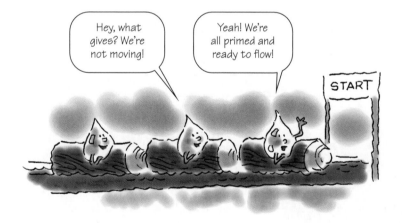

> **Pep talk**
>
> " There are admirable potentialities in every human being. Believe in your strength and your youth. Learn to repeat endlessly to yourself, 'It all depends on me.' "
> —Andre Gide

Hit or miss

Mark each statement about electronic infusion devices with a "T" for "True" and an "F" for "False."

_____ 1. Electronic devices such as pumps aren't routinely used because they aren't as reliable as standard infusion sets.

_____ 2. Electronic devices such as pumps help regulate the rate and volume of infusions.

_____ 3. A change in the infusion rate will trigger an alarm.

_____ 4. It's unnecessary to disengage an electronic infusion device when infiltration occurs.

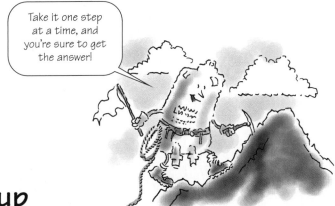

Take it one step at a time, and you're sure to get the answer!

Starting lineup

Reorder the steps below to show the correct sequence for setting up and running an infusion pump.

Prime and place the I.V. tubing, making sure to flush all the air out of the tubing before connecting it to the patient.
Attach the pump to the I.V. pole, and then insert the administration spike into the I.V. container.
Set the appropriate controls to the desired infusion rate or volume.
Fill the drip chamber completely to prevent air bubbles from entering the tubing, and clamp the tubing while the pump door is open.
Check the patency of the venous access device, watch for infiltration, and monitor the accuracy of the infusion rate.
Place the infusion pump on the same side of the bed as the I.V. setup and the intended venipuncture site.

Winner's circle

Although vein selection for a venipuncture device depends on several variables, three types of veins are most commonly used. Circle the most commonly used veins on the illustration below.

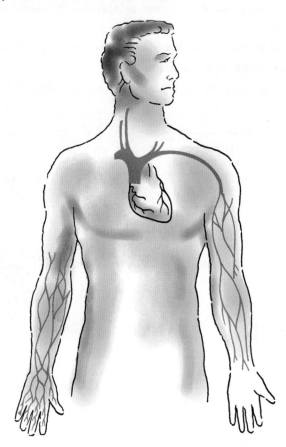

Strikeout

These statements provide general guidelines for selecting an appropriate vein for peripheral venipuncture. Cross out the incorrect statements.

1. Usually, the most prominent veins are the best choices.

2. You should never select a vein in an edematous or impaired arm.

3. You should never select a vein in the arm closest to an area that's surgically compromised.

4. You should never select a vein in the affected arm of a patient following a stroke.

5. You should try to select a vein in the patient's dominant arm or hand whenever possible.

6. For subsequent venipunctures, you should select sites below the previously used or injured vein.

7. You should make sure to rotate access sites.

Power stretch

Stretch your knowledge of venipuncture vein sites by first unscrambling the words on the left to reveal some commonly used veins. Then draw a line from the box to the major advantages or disadvantages to using it. Note that some veins will match up with more than one set of advantages or disadvantages.

HEALCICP

— — — — — — — —

GAITLID

— — — — — — — —

PLEATACRAM

— — — — — — — — — —

SCABLII

— — — — — — —

ABLECATNUIT

— — — — — — — — — — —

A. May be used for short-term therapy and when other means aren't available

B. Large vein that readily accepts large-gauge needles, excellent for venipuncture, doesn't impair mobility

C. Straight, strong vein that takes large-gauge needle easily

D. Difficult to dislodge from site, bones around site often act like a splint

E. Requires splinting fingers with a tongue blade, may be uncomfortable

F. May be small and scarred if blood has been drawn frequently from this site

G. Large vein that facilitates drawing blood, sometimes used in an emergency or as a last resort

H. Device insertion here commonly painful because of large number of nerve endings in hand

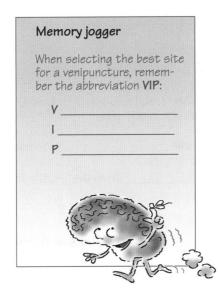

Memory jogger

When selecting the best site for a venipuncture, remember the abbreviation **VIP**:

V _____

I _____

P _____

I'm warning you: If you're not in shape, you won't make the cut!

Hit or miss

Mark each of these statements about vein choices for peripheral venipunctures with a "T" for "True" and an "F" for "False."

_____ 1. Generally, the deep veins in the dorsum of the hand and forearm are the best choices.

_____ 2. The dorsum of the forearm has long, straight veins with fairly large diameters, which makes them convenient for introducing large-bore needles and long I.V. catheters used in prolonged I.V. therapy.

_____ 3. Veins of the hand and forearm are suitable for most drugs and solutions.

_____ 4. The metacarpal and basilic veins in the upper arm are more suitable for irritating drugs and solutions with high osmolarity.

_____ 5. The dorsum of the hand is well-supplied with small, superficial veins that can easily dilate and usually accommodate a catheter.

_____ 6. The dorsal venous network (on the dorsal portion of the foot) may be suitable to use for infants and toddlers; however, it's difficult to find a vein if edema is present.

_____ 7. When leg or foot veins must be used, the saphenous vein of the inner aspect of the ankle and the veins of the dorsal foot network are best—but only as a last resort.

_____ 8. Venous access in the lower extremities carries a deceased risk of thrombophlebitis.

_____ 9. Use of a venous access device in an upper arm can compromise the use of sites distal to the upper arm.

_____ 10. Upper arm veins are sometimes difficult to locate in obese patients and in those with shorter arms such as children.

Batter's box

Watch out for curveballs when completing the missing information on differentiating arteries from veins below. Remember to use each option only once.

Arteries are located deep in _____ and _____ . Arteries contain
                              1   2

_____ red blood that flows _____ from the heart, veins contain
        3   4

_____ red blood that flows _____ the heart. If you
        5   6

_____ an artery, the blood _____ from the site. Only veins have
        7   8

_____ ; they're usually only apparent in long, straight _____ veins
        9   10

that have good tone. A _____ valve will appear as a painless knot within a vein.
                              11

Options

A. arm

B. away

C. bright

D. dark

E. muscles

F. pulsates

G. puncture

H. sclerosed

I. soft tissues

J. toward

K. valves

■ Finish line

Understanding the anatomy of skin and veins can help you locate appropriate venipuncture sites and perform venipunctures with minimal patient discomfort. Identify the major skin and vein structures pictured below.

Layers of the skin

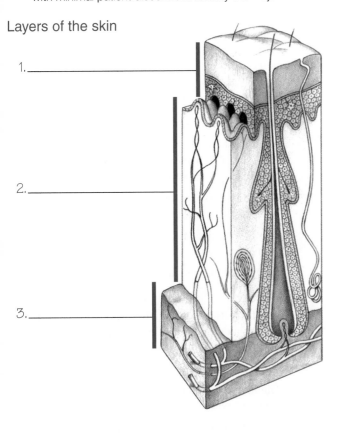

1._____

2._____

3._____

Layers of veins

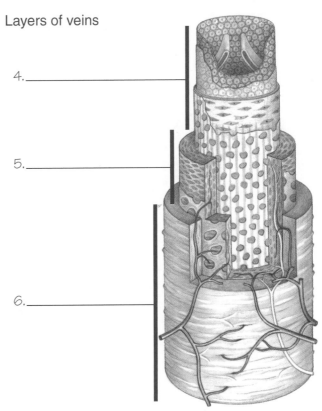

4._____

5._____

6._____

■ Power stretch

Stretch your knowledge of skin and vein layers a little further by first unscrambling the words on the left to reveal the layer names. Then draw a line from each box to its corresponding characteristics on the right.

IUCTNA DAEIM

— — — — — — — — — — —

MIDSER

— — — — — —

AINTUC DATIVNTEAI

— — — — — —

— — — — — — — — — —

DREMPISIE

— — — — — — — — —

AUSNUSCBOTEU IUSETS

— — — — — — — — — — —

— — — — — —

UTAICN IMAITN

— — — — — — — — — — —

A. Top layer that forms a protective covering for the skin, having varied thickness in different parts of body

B. Valves in this layer are located in semilunar folds of the endothelium

C. Site of superficial veins

D. Inner elastic endothelial lining made up of smooth, flat cells, which allow blood cells and platelets to flow smoothly through the blood vessel

E. Connective tissue that surrounds and supports the vessels and holds it together

F. Highly sensitive and vascular because it contains many capillaries

G. Composed of muscular and elastic tissue

H. Located below the two layers of skin

I. Location of vasoconstrictor and vasodilator nerve fibers that stimulate veins to contract and relax

J. Location of thousands of nerves, which react to temperature, touch, pressure, and pain

K. Thickness and amount of connective tissue decrease with age, resulting in fragile veins

L. Contains about 25 layers of cells with bacteria in the top five layers

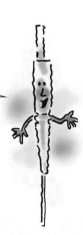

It helps to be thoroughly familiar with the ins and outs of skin and vein layers—if you get my point!

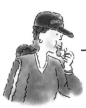

Coaching session
Vein selection guidelines

All things being equal, choose a vein that's:
- distal (unless the solution is very irritating, such as potassium chloride)
- full and pliable
- long enough to accommodate the length of the intended catheter (about 1")
- large enough to allow blood flow around the catheter (to minimize venous lumen irritation).
  Don't choose a vein that's:
- bruised
- tender
- phlebitic
- over a flexion area (such as the wrist or antecubital fossa).
  Some veins are best to avoid, including:
- legs (circulation may be compromised)
- inner wrist and arm (they're small and uncomfortable)
- affected arm of a mastectomy patient
- arm with an arteriovenous shunt or fistula
- arm being treated for thrombosis or cellulitis
- arm that has experienced trauma (such as burns or scarring from surgery).

■ Strikeout

When selecting a venous access device, it's usually best to go with the shortest length and smallest diameter that allows for proper administration of the therapy. Cross out the statements that aren't a consideration when choosing a venous access device.

1. Time of day when venipuncture or infusion will occur

2. Length of therapy or time the device will stay in place

3. Type of therapy

4. Type of procedure or surgery to be preformed

5. Patient's age and activity level

6. Patient's blood type

7. Patient's privacy

8. Type of solution used

9. Condition of veins

■ Hit or miss

Mark each of these statements about venous access devices with a "T" for "True" or an "F" for "False."

_____ 1. The two most commonly used devices are plastic catheter sets and winged needle sets.

_____ 2. As a rule, plastic catheters allow more patient movement and activity and are less prone to infiltration; however, they're more difficult to insert.

_____ 3. An over-the-needle catheter is the most commonly used device for peripheral I.V. therapy.

_____ 4. Over-the-needle catheters consist of a plastic outer tube and an inner needle that extends just beyond the catheter.

_____ 5. The over-the-needle catheters used for routine venipunctures are available in lengths of 1″ and 2″, with gauges ranging from 14 to 26.

_____ 6. The catheter portion of an over-the-needle catheter set is typically left in place for 2 to 3 days, depending on the facility's policy and procedures.

_____ 7. A winged needle catheter has a long, large-bore tubing between the catheter and hub and is especially useful for delicate veins and for intermittent or one-time medication administration when I.V. access isn't otherwise needed.

_____ 8. Winged needle catheters are commonly called *butterfly needles*; they have no hub and lie flat on the skin, making taping easy.

_____ 9. Butterfly needles are commonly used for I.V. bolus injections as well as for patients with sclerosed veins and those who require long-term infusion of I.V. fluids or medications.

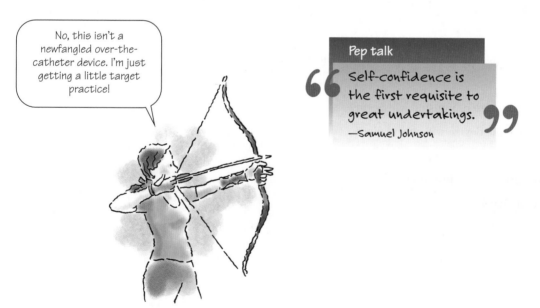

No, this isn't a newfangled over-the-catheter device. I'm just getting a little target practice!

Pep talk

❝ Self-confidence is the first requisite to great undertakings. ❞
—Samuel Johnson

You make the call

Identify the two major types of venous access devices pictured here. Then fill in the advantages and disadvantages of each one on the lines provided.

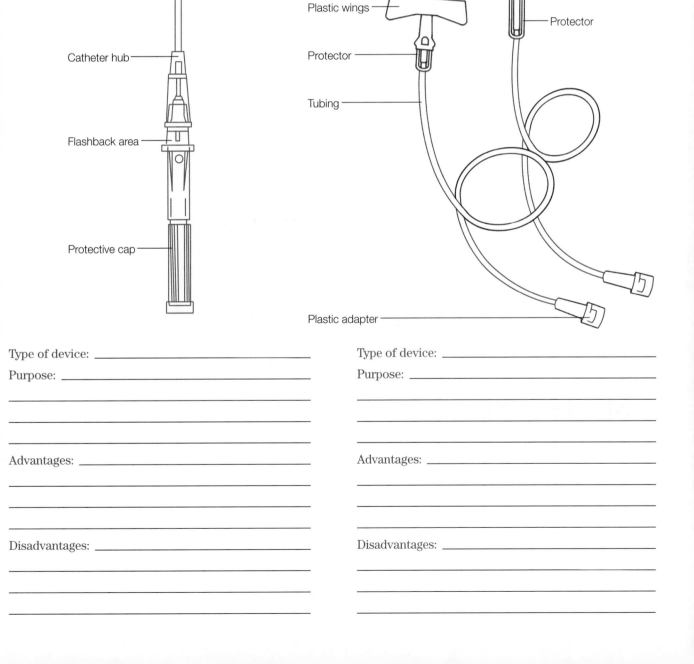

1.
- Needle
- Catheter
- Catheter hub
- Flashback area
- Protective cap

2.
- Needle
- Plastic wings
- Protector
- Tubing
- Needle
- Protector
- Plastic adapter

Type of device: _____

Purpose: _____

_____

_____

_____

Advantages: _____

_____

_____

_____

Disadvantages: _____

_____

_____

_____

Type of device: _____

Purpose: _____

_____

_____

_____

Advantages: _____

_____

_____

_____

Disadvantages: _____

_____

_____

_____

Match point

Use of the correct gauge needle depends on the patient's age and condition as well as the type of infusion. Match each gauge on the left with its typical uses and nursing considerations on the right.

Gauge
1. 16 _____
2. 18 _____
3. 20 _____
4. 22 _____
5. 24 or 26 _____

Typical uses and nursing considerations

A. Used for toddlers, children, adolescents, and adults (especially elderly adults); commonly used for most I.V. infusions; is easier to insert into smaller veins

B. Used for older children, adolescents, and adults; used to administer of blood and blood components and other viscous infusions; is routinely used postoperatively; can cause painful insertion; requires a large vein

C. Used for adolescents and adults; used in major surgery or trauma situations, typically whenever large amounts of fluids must be infused rapidly; can cause painful insertion; requires a large vein

D. Used for neonates, infants, toddlers, school-age children, adolescents, and adults (especially elderly adults); suitable for most infusions, but flow rates are slower; used in extremely small veins (small veins of fingers or veins of inner arms); can be difficult to insert through tough skin

E. Used for children, adolescents, and adults; suitable for most I.V. infusions, blood, blood components, and other viscous infusions; is commonly used

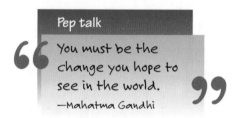

Pep talk

" You must be the change you hope to see in the world.
—Mahatma Gandhi "

Mind sprints

Six factors help determine how long a venous access device can remain in place.
See if you can name them all in 2 minutes or less.

- _____
- _____
- _____
- _____
- _____
- _____

Cross-training

Infuse yourself with even more knowledge of venipunctures and venous access devices by solving this crossword puzzle.

Across

2. Stabilizing device used in venipunctures (two words)

7. Device that impedes venous flow by trapping blood in veins

9. Common antimicrobial cleaning solution

12. Type of drug used to reduce the discomfort associated with venipuncture

13. Slanted or angled edge of a needle

14. Measurement by which needles and catheters are described

Down

1. Handheld device that uses electric current to deliver lidocaine and epinephrine to numb the skin

3. Other name for a winged needle catheter (two words)

4. Type of side-by-side catheter used for simultaneous infusion of two incompatible solutions (two words)

5. Chamber inside catheter where blood return collects

6. Intermittent infusion device used to maintain venous access (two words)

8. Type of access cap placed over catheter's adapter end that allows for an add-on infusion (two words)

10. One of two key ingredients in antimicrobial solution that also includes iodine

11. Over-the-_____ catheter

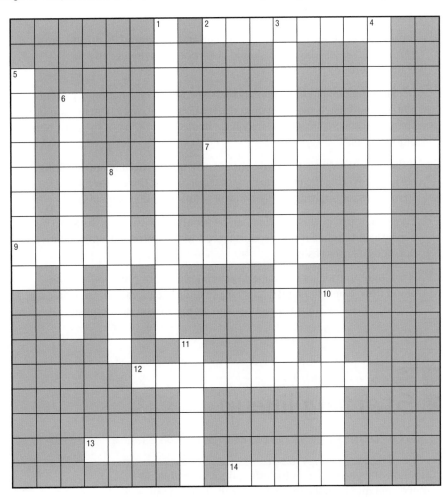

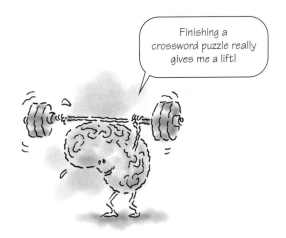

Finishing a crossword puzzle really gives me a lift!

■ Strikeout

A tourniquet helps to dilate a vein in preparation of a venipuncture. Cross out the incorrect term or phrase in these statements about tourniquets.

1. A properly distended vein should appear and feel round, firm, and partially filled with blood. It should also rebound when gently compressed.

2. Because the amount of trapped blood depends on circulation, a patient who's hypotensive, overly hydrated, very cold, or experiencing vasomotor changes (as in septic shock) may have inadequate filling of the peripheral blood vessels.

3. If the patient's skin is cold; you should warm it by rubbing and stroking his arm; covering the entire arm with warm, moist towels for 5 to 10 minutes; or applying a 10% menthol solution to the skin surface.

4. The ideal tourniquet is one that can be secured easily, turns the skin beneath and around it purple, doesn't roll into a thin band, stays relatively flat, and releases easily.

5. A too-tight tourniquet can impede arterial blood flow, impede venous blood flow, cause bruising (especially in elderly patients whose veins are fragile), cause an allergic reaction, and obliterate the radial pulse.

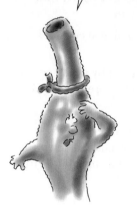

I'm not usually this pumped up. I think my tourniquet has been in place about 30 seconds too long.

■ Starting lineup

Put these steps in proper order to describe the safe way of applying a tourniquet.

Holding one end on top of the other, lift and stretch the tourniquet and tuck the top tail under the bottom tail—without loosening the tourniquet.	
Place the tourniquet under the patient's arm, about 6″ (15 cm) above the venipuncture site.	
Bring the ends of the tourniquet together, placing one on top of the other.	
Place the arm on the middle of the tourniquet.	
Tie the tourniquet smoothly and snugly, being careful not to pinch the patient's skin or pull his arm hair.	

■ Boxing match

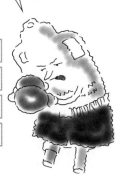

Is a technical knockout an acceptable form of local anesthetic? (Just kidding!)

Cleaning solutions and local anesthetics are used to prepare the access site for a venipuncture. Fill in the answers to the clues below by using all the syllables in the box. The number of syllables for each answer is shown in parentheses. Use each syllable only once.

A	CAINE	CHLOR	DER	DINE	DINE	DINE
DO	DONE	E	GE	HEX	I	I
I	I	LI	MAL	NAL	NE	O
O	ON	PHO	PHRINE	PI	PO	RE
SIC	SIS	TO	TRANS	VI		

1. A 2% solution of this is commonly used to clean the skin   (4) _ _ _ _ _ _ _ _ _ _ _ _ _

2. A thin coat of a 10% solution of this cleans the skin   (6) _ _ _ _ _ _ _ _ — _ _ _ _ _ _

3. Some antimicrobial solutions contain a 2% tincture of this ingredient   (3) _ _ _ _ _ _

4. Often given as an injectable local anesthetic   (3) _ _ _ _ _ _ _ _ _

5. Type of cream used to numb the skin   (7) _ _ _ _ _ _ _ _ _ _ _
_ _ _ _ _ _ _ _ _

6. Handheld device that uses electrodes to deliver numbing agents   (6) _ _ _ _ _ _ _ _ _ _ _ _ _

7. One of the drugs used in #6, available in a 1:100,000 solution   (4) _ _ _ _ _ _ _ _ _ _ _

■ You make the call

Identify the procedure pictured below, and briefly explain its relevance to peripheral I.V. therapy.

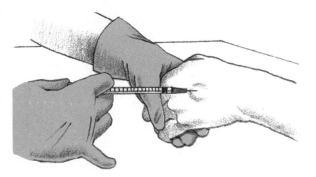

Procedure: _____

Relevance: _____
_____
_____
_____
_____
_____

■ ■
■ Strikeout

Cross out the incorrect statements about giving a lidocaine injection.

1. Administering a local anesthetic such as lidocaine requires using a U-100 insulin syringe with a 27G needle.

2. Lidocaine is best administered directly into the vein, where it can take immediate effect.

3. To perform the injection, you should first clean the venipuncture site, and then insert the needle next to the vein, introducing about one-third of it into the skin at a 30-degree angle.

4. After inserting the needle, you should immediately aspirate to check for a blood return. If blood appears, withdraw the needle and begin again.

5. Once the needle is correctly placed, you should quickly inject the lidocaine until a small wheal appears.

6. A lidocaine injection should keep the skin numb for at least 1 hour.

■ ■
■ Batter's box

Fill in the blanks with the answer options below to complete these statements about vein stabilization. Use each option only once.

Stabilizing the vein helps ensure a successful venipuncture the first time and decreases the

chance of _____ . If the tip of the venous access device repeatedly probes a
          1

_____ vein wall, it can nick the vein and cause it to leak blood. A nicked
          2

vein can't be reused immediately, which results in finding a new venipuncture site and

causing the patient additional _____ .
                                    3

    To stabilize the vein, _____ the skin and hold it _____ ,
                              4   5

and then lightly press it with your fingertip about 1½″ (3.5 cm) from the insertion site.

Avoid retouching the prepared site or you'll _____ it. The vein should feel
                                                  6

round, firm, fully _____ , and resilient, if it returns to its original position
                        7

and appears larger than it did before applying the tourniquet, it's adequately

_____ .
          8

    To help prevent the vein from _____ , apply adequate traction to the
                                      9

vein with your _____ hand to hold the skin and vein in place.
                     10

Options
A. bruising
B. discomfort
C. distended
D. engorged
E. moving
F. nondominant
G. recontaminate
H. rolling
I. stretch
J. taut

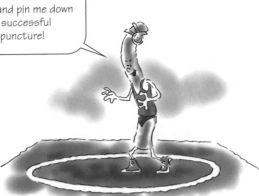

You'll need to learn a few good maneuvers to stabilize and pin me down for a successful venipuncture!

Match point

To help ensure a successful venipuncture, you need to stabilize the patient's vein by stretching the skin and holding it taut. Match the vein on the left with the stretching technique on the right.

Vein

1. Antecubital fossa _____

2. Basilic vein at outer arm _____

3. Cephalic vein above the wrist _____

4. Dorsum of foot _____

5. Inner arm _____

6. Inner aspect of wrist _____

7. Metacarpal (hand) veins _____

8. Saphenous vein of ankle _____

9. Scalp _____

Stretching technique

A. Stretch the patient's hand and wrist downward, and hold the skin taut with your thumb.

B. Stretch the patient's fist laterally downward, and immobilize the skin with the thumb of your other hand.

C. Hold the skin taut with your thumb and forefinger.

D. Have the patient flex his elbow. While standing behind the flexed arm, retract the skin away from the site, and anchor the vein with your thumb. Alternatively, rotate the patient's extended lower arm inward, and approach the vein from behind the arm.

E. Anchor the patient's vein with your thumb above the wrist.

F. Extend the patient's foot downward and inward. Anchor the vein with your thumb, about 2″ to 3″ (5 to 7.5 cm) below the ankle.

G. Extend the patient's open hand backward from the wrist. Anchor the vein with your thumb below the insertion site.

H. Pull the patient's foot downward. Anchor the vein with your thumb, about 2″ to 3″ below the vein (usually near the toes).

I. Have the patient extend his arm completely. Anchor the skin with your thumb, about 2″ to 3″ below the vein.

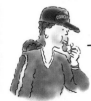

Coaching session
Advancing a winged infusion set

If you're using a winged infusion set, advance the needle as carefully as possible and hold it in place. Release the tourniquet, slightly open the administration set clamp, and check for free flow or infiltration. Next, tape the infusion set in place, using the wings as an anchor to prevent catheter movement, which could cause irritation and phlebitis.

■ Starting lineup

Once you've prepared the venipuncture site, you're ready to position the venous access device for insertion. Put these statements in the correct order to indicate the proper positioning and insertion technique.

Advance the device to at least one-half its length, at which point you should see blood in the flashback chamber.
Examine the device. If the edge isn't smooth, discard the device and obtain another one.
Grasp the plastic hub with your dominant hand and remove the cover.
Tell the patient that you're about to insert the device, and ask him to remain still and refrain from pulling away.
Insert the device, bevel up, through the skin and into the vein at a 5- to 15-degree angle (deeper veins require a wider angle).
Lower the hub (the distal portion of the adapter) until it's almost parallel to the skin.

■ Hit or miss

Mark each of these statements about inserting and advancing an over-the-needle venous access device with a "T" for "True" or an "F" for "False."

_____ 1. You will always hear a "pop" or sense a release when the device enters the vein.

_____ 2. To advance the catheter into the vein before starting an infusion, you should first release the tourniquet.

_____ 3. Advancing the needle as well as the catheter ensures that the device is completely in the vein.

_____ 4. Applying digital pressure to the catheter while removing the inner needle minimizes the risk of blood exposure.

_____ 5. You should always use aseptic technique while attaching the I.V. tubing or flushing the inserted device with saline solution.

_____ 6. To advance the device while an infusion is running, you should reduce the flow rate and push the needle forward into the vein.

_____ 7. Advancing the catheter while infusing I.V. fluids doesn't increase the risk of infection.

_____ 8. After the access site has been successfully inserted and securely taped, you should clean the skin, cover the access site with a transparent dressing (or the dressing used by your facility), dispose of the needle, and regulate the flow rate.

_____ 9. You should always dispose of the inner needle in a nonpermeable receptacle.

You make the call

Identify the device pictured below, and briefly describe why it's used.

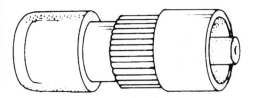

Device: _____

Reason for use: _____

_____

_____

_____

_____

> Just killing a little time between infusions. If you'd like to join in, I can always use another steady-ender.

Mind sprints

An intermittent infusion device maintains venous access for intermittent use when continuous I.V. infusion isn't ordered. In 2 minutes or less, list five major benefits associated with its use.

- _____
- _____
- _____
- _____
- _____

Train your brain

Sound out this puzzle to discover an important fact about medication infusion.

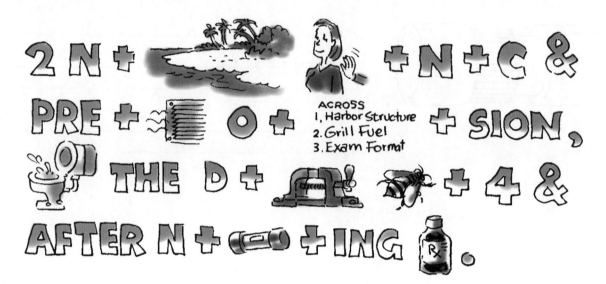

ACROSS
1. Harbor Structure
2. Grill Fuel
3. Exam Format

Batter's box

Flushing an I.V. line with saline solution expels air from the equipment and allows you to maintain venous access. For additional information, fill in the blanks below with the answer options provided.

If the patient feels a _____ sensation as you inject saline solution,
                              1

_____ the injection and check the _____ placement.
        2   3

If it's in the _____ , inject the solution at a _____
                    4   5

rate to minimize _____ .
                        6

Options
A. burning
B. catheter
C. irritation
D. slower
E. stop
F. vein

■ Starting lineup

Sometimes you'll need to insert a venous access device into a deep vein when a superficial vein isn't available. Put these steps in the correct sequence to explain how this is done.

After putting on gloves, palpate the area with your fingertips until you feel the vein.	
Clean the skin over the vein with a cleaning solution, swiping in a side-to-side motion.	
Remove the tourniquet and inner needle, and advance the catheter.	
Insert the device about one-half to two-thirds its length at a 15-degree angle to the skin.	
Look for blood in the flashback chamber.	
Aim the device directly over the vein, and stretch the skin with your fingertips.	

■ Strikeout

Cross out the incorrect statements about collecting a blood sample while performing a venipuncture.

1. To collect blood, you'll need all of the following equipment: one or more evacuated tubes, a 26G needleless system, an appropriate-size syringe without a needle, and a protective pad.

2. You should leave the tourniquet tied until after the syringe is attached and the appropriate amount of blood is withdrawn.

3. You should wait 10 minutes after blood collection before attaching a saline lock or I.V. tubing. You should then regulate the flow rate and stabilize the device.

4. After attaching the needleless system to the syringe with the collected blood, you should transfer the blood into the evacuated tubes.

A saline flush can be so refreshing after blood collection!

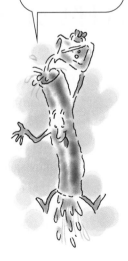

■ You make the call

If you use tape to secure the venous access device, you'll probably use one of the methods shown here. Name the method and describe the procedure in the blank spaces provided.

1.

2.

3.

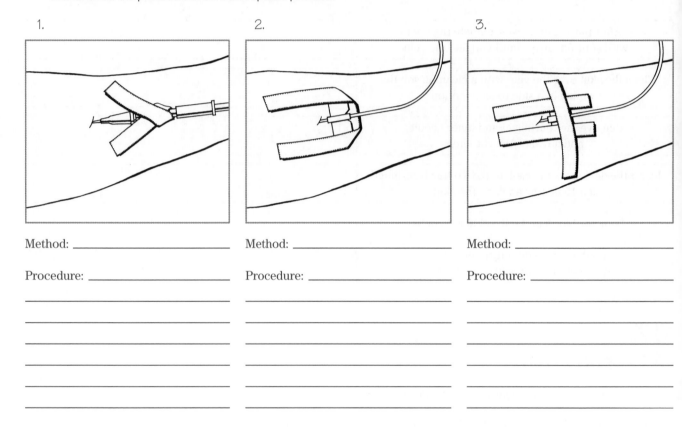

Method: _____

Procedure: _____

_____

_____

_____

_____

_____

Method: _____

Procedure: _____

_____

_____

_____

_____

_____

Method: _____

Procedure: _____

_____

_____

_____

_____

_____

■ Hit or miss

Mark each statement about securing venous access devices with "T" for "True" and an "F" for "False."

_____ 1. To secure a venous access device, you should use sterile tape or a transparent dressing.

_____ 2. Standard taping methods include the chevron, U, and 12-point methods.

_____ 3. You should always use as little tape as possible, and make sure the tape ends meet.

_____ 4. Removing hair around the access area improves visibility and reduces pain when the tape is removed.

_____ 5. Removing hair around the access area should be done with a razor.

_____ 6. You shouldn't let tape cover the patient's skin too far beyond the infusion device's entry site.

_____ 7. Swelling and redness are common with taping and indicate that the dressing is secure.

_____ 8. It's best to use paper tape for dressings because it's easy to remove.

Mind sprints

Think fast! In 2 minutes or less, list five advantages to using a transparent semipermeable dressing.

- _____
- _____
- _____
- _____
- _____

You make the call

Using the spaces provided, identify the procedure illustrated below and explain why it's done.

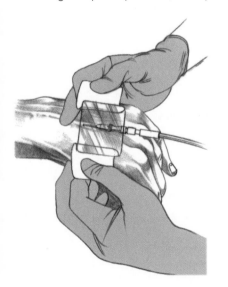

Procedure: _____

Why it's done: _____

_____

_____

_____

_____

Pep talk

"Practice, which some regard as a chore, should be approached as just about the most pleasant recreation ever devised.

—Babe Didrikson"

■ Jumble gym

Use the clues to help you unscramble words related to securing venous access devices. Then use the circled letters to answer the question posed.

Question: To determine whether a patient requires an arm board with a venous access device, you need to observe for stoppage of I.V. flow while he performs what maneuvers?

1. Applied over the affected limb of confused or very active patients (especially children) to cut down on amount of tape needed to hold infusion device in place

T E C S H T R   E N T _ _ _ ◯ _ _ _   _ _ ◯ _

2. Applied on affected limb to secure venous access device positioning and prevent unnecessary motion that could cause infiltration or inflammation; may be considered a form of restraint in some states

R M A   R O B A D _ _ _   _ ◯ _ ◯ _

3. Applied over site to keep venous access device clean, dry, and always visible for inspection

E E M I E S L P E R A M B   N T R S R E A A N T P   S S D R G E I N
_ _ _ ◯ _ _ _ ◯ _ _ _ _ _   _ _ _ _ _ _ ◯ _ _ _ _
_ _ _ _ _ _ ◯ _

4. The act of bending a limb or joint

N I X F E L O ◯ _ _ _ _ ◯ _

5. Forced movement from a previously fixed position; can occur with catheters or dressings

G L I S T E D M O N D _ _ _ _ _ _ _ ◯ _ _ ◯ _

6. The act of preventing movement or motion to promote healing

M A I L Z O N B I T O I M I _ ◯ _ ◯ _ _ _ _ _ _ _ _ _ _

Answer: _ _ _ _ _   _ _   _ _ _ _ _ _

■ Mind sprints

You must document several key pieces of information whenever you start an I.V. line. Time yourself, and see how many items you can list in 2 minutes.

- _____
- _____
- _____
- _____
- _____

- _____
- _____
- _____
- _____
- _____

■ Batter's box

Once a peripheral infusion is started, the focus shifts to providing routine care. Complete the statements by using the answer options below.

Routine care measures help prevent _____ . They also give you an
                                            1

opportunity to observe the site for signs of _____ and _____ —
                                                      2   3

two of the most common complications. One important way to cut down on the risk of

complications is to always wear _____ and to wash your _____
                                          4   5

whenever you work near the _____ site.
                                    6

> **Options**
> A. complications
> B. gloves
> C. hands
> D. infection
> E. inflammation
> F. venipuncture

■ Starting lineup

Put these steps in the correct sequence to explain how to change a peripheral I.V. dressing.

If you don't detect complications, hold the needle or catheter at the hub and carefully clean around the site with an alcohol swab or another approved solution. Work in a swiping motion to avoid introducing pathogens into the cleaned are. Allow the site to dry completely.	
If you detect any sign of complications, apply pressure to the area with a sterile gauze pad and remove the catheter or needle, maintain pressure until bleeding stops, and then apply an adhesive bandage. Using new equipment, insert the I.V. access at another site.	
Wash your hands and put on sterile gloves.	
Assess the venipuncture site for signs of infection, infiltration, and thrombophlebitis.	
Retape the device and apply a transparent semipermeable dressing, or apply gauze and secure it.	
Hold the needle or catheter in place with your nondominant hand to prevent movement or dislodgment that could lead to infection, then gently remove the tape and the dressing.	

Strikeout

Cross out all of the incorrect statements about routine care procedures.

1. The equipment you'll need for a routine dressing change includes an alcohol swab or other approved solution, adhesive bandage, sterile 2″ × 2″ gauze pad or transparent semipermeable dressing, 1″ sterile adhesive tape, and sterile gloves.

2. To avoid microbial growth, you shouldn't allow an I.V. solution container to hang for more than 48 hours.

3. Before changing an I.V. container, check the new one for cracks, leaks, and other damage and check the solution for discoloration, turbidity, and particulates.

4. You should always preset the flow rate before spiking and hanging a new I.V. container to save time.

5. Most facilities dictate changing I.V. administration sets on a daily basis (for a primary infusion line) and whenever contamination is suspected.

6. I.V. sites are usually rotated every 72 hours as a standard of care.

7. The entire I.V. system should be replaced if the patient has signs of thrombophlebitis, cellulitis, or I.V. related bacteremia.

Power stretch

Stretch your knowledge of special I.V. procedures that you may be asked to perform or assist with by first unscrambling the words on the left. Then draw a line from the box to the definition or characteristics at right.

ITAIDEVD
OINNSIUF

_ _ _ _ _ _ _ _

_ _ _ _ _ _ _ _

VENI
IOCTDSSNIE

_ _ _ _

_ _ _ _ _ _ _ _ _ _

A. Uses an add-a-line administration set

B. Also called a *venous cutdown*

C. Requires making a small incision in the skin over the vein

D. Also called a *piggyback infusion*

E. May be needed when usual venipuncture techniques become impossible due to obesity, collapsed veins, sclerosis, or vasoconstriction from massive, rapid blood loss

This exercise really stretches your understanding of special I.V. situations.

Hit or miss

Mark each statement about the special needs of pediatric patients receiving I.V. infusions with a "T" for "True" and an "F" for "False."

_____ 1. The veins of an infant or toddler are close to the surface, making them fairly easy to access.

_____ 2. A premature infant has less subcutaneous fat than a full-term infant, so his veins are more prominent.

_____ 3. The best I.V. insertion sites in an infant are in the dorsum of the hand, feet antecubital fossa, and scalp.

_____ 4. An infant's scalp has a small supply of veins and, therefore, it is usually used as a last resort in those under age 6 months.

_____ 5. In toddlers, the dorsum of the hand offers the best site for venipuncture.

_____ 6. Because scalp veins can resemble arteries, you should always palpate to ensure you have a vein and not an artery before performing a venipuncture on a scalp vein.

_____ 7. You'll feel a palpable pulse with a vein, not an artery.

_____ 8. When necessary, you should use a clove-hitch or mummy restraint to keep an infant still during a venipuncture.

_____ 9. Tourniquets and rubber bands can be used on infants but not on older children.

_____ 10. The preferred venous access device for infants and young children is a large-bore over-the-needle catheter (also called a *scalp vein catheter*).

_____ 11. Use extra tape over the I.V. site and surrounding area to stabilize the site and ensure adhesion.

_____ 12. If an emergency intraosseous infusion is needed to provide resuscitative fluid, medication, or blood, a 16G or 19G straight needle is placed directly into the medullary cavity of bone (typically the distal end of the femur or the proximal or distal ends of the tibia).

Finish line

Identify the scalp veins most commonly used for venipuncture in infants.

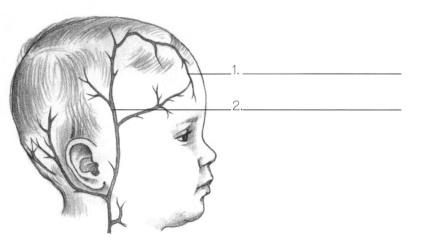

1. _____

2. _____

■ Strikeout

Elderly patients also pose a particular challenge during peripheral I.V. infusion. Cross out the incorrect statements.

1. Veins in elderly patients are typically not prominent and are difficult to see.

2. An elderly patient's skin is less resistant to puncture than that of a younger patient and is therefore easier to access for venipuncture.

3. Because an elderly patient's tissues are looser than a younger patient's, stabilizing veins is sometimes more difficult.

4. The thickness and amount of connective tissue in the outer layer of veins tend to decrease with age; therefore, the veins become more fragile.

5. It's best to perform a venipuncture slowly on an older patient to avoid excessive bruising.

6. A smaller-gauge needle (such as a 24G ¾″ needle) is commonly easier to insert in an elderly person.

7. You should keep the tourniquet on longer than usual with an elderly patient to ensure the vein stays distended during venipuncture.

8. An elderly patient's veins typically appear tortuous because of the increased transparency and decreased elasticity of the skin.

9. The veins also appear large because venous pressure is inadequate.

10. To help stabilize a vein for insertion, stretch the skin proximal to the insertion site and anchor it firmly with your nondominant hand.

■ Team up!

Local and systemic complications can arise from the venous access device, the infusion, or the medication being administered. Indicate whether these complications are local or systemic by putting them under the respective headings.

Local   Systemic

_____   _____
_____   _____
_____   _____
_____   _____
_____   _____
_____   _____
_____   _____
_____   _____
_____   _____

- Allergic reaction
- Catheter dislodgment (extravasation)
- Cellulitis
- Circulatory overload
- Embolism
- Hematoma
- Infiltration
- Nerve, tendon, or ligament damage
- Occlusion
- Phlebitis
- Septicemia
- Severed or fractured catheter
- Thrombophlebitis
- Thrombosis
- Vasovagal reaction
- Vein irritation or pain at I.V. site
- Venous spasm

■ Match point

Match each complication on the left with its signs and symptoms on the right.

Complication

1. Phlebitis _____
2. Infiltration _____
3. Catheter dislodgment _____
4. Occlusion _____
5. Vein irritation or pain at I.V. site _____
6. Severed catheter _____
7. Hematoma _____
8. Venous spasm _____
9. Thrombosis _____
10. Thrombophlebitis _____
11. Nerve, tendon, or ligament damage _____
12. Circulatory overload _____
13. Systemic infection _____
14. Embolism _____
15. Allergic reaction _____

Signs and symptoms

A. Severe discomfort; reddened, swollen, or hardened vein

B. Discomfort, jugular vein engorgement, respiratory distress, increased blood pressure, crackles, large positive fluid balance

C. Pain during infusion, possible blanching if vasospasm occurs; red skin over vein during infusion; rapidly developing signs of phlebitis

D. Tenderness at tip of infusion device and above, redness at tip of catheter and along vein, puffy area over vein, vein hard on palpation, elevated temperature

E. Leakage from catheter shaft

F. No increase in flow rate when I.V. container is raised, blood backup in line, discomfort at insertion site

G. Swelling at and around I.V. site (possibly along entire limb); discomfort, burning, or pain at site; feeling of tightness; decreased skin temperature and blanching at site; absent backflow of blood; slower flow rate

H. Fever, chills, and malaise for no apparent reason; contaminated I.V. site (usually with no visible signs of infection at site)

I. Pain along vein, sluggish flow rate when clamp is completely open, blanched skin over vein

J. Itching, tearing eyes and runny nose, bronchospasm, wheezing, urticarial rash, edema at I.V. site anaphylactic reaction (within minutes or up to 1 hour after exposure)

K. Extreme pain (similar to electric shock when nerve is contracted), numbness and muscle contraction, delayed effects (paralysis, numbness, and deformity)

L. Respiratory distress, unequal breath sounds, weak pulse, increased central venous pressure, decreased blood pressure, confusion, disorientation, loss of consciousness

M. Catheter partly backed out of vein, infusate infiltrating

N. Tenderness at venipuncture site, bruising around site, inability to advance or flush I.V. line

O. Painful, reddened, and swollen vein; sluggish or stopped I.V. flow

■ Mind sprints

In 1 minute or less, list four important pieces of information you're required to document when complications develop during peripheral I.V. therapy.

- _____
- _____
- _____
- _____

■ Starting lineup

Put the following statements in correct order to explain how to discontinue a peripheral I.V. infusion.

Dispose of used venipuncture equipment, tubing, and solution in the designated receptacles.	
After putting on gloves, lift the tape from the skin to expose the insertion site. Avoid manipulating the device to prevent organisms from entering the skin and to prevent discomfort.	
Apply a sterile 2″ × 2″ dressing directly over the insertion site, and then quickly remove the device.	
Document the time of removal, the catheter length and integrity, and the condition of the site. Also record how the patient tolerated the procedure and any nursing interventions.	
Tell the patient to restrict his activity for about 10 minutes and to leave the dressing in place for at least 8 hours. Advise him to apply warm, moist packs if tenderness lingers at the site.	
Maintain direct pressure on the site for several minutes, and then tape a dressing over it, being careful not to encircle the limb. If possible, hold the limb upright for about 5 minutes to decrease venous pressure.	

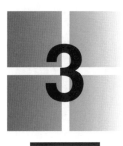

3

Central venous therapy

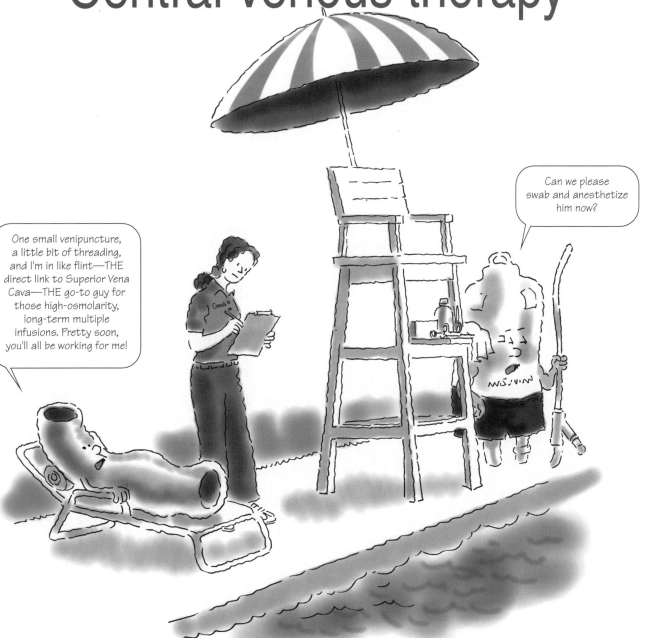

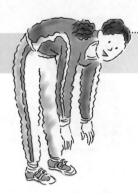

Central venous therapy review

Benefits

- Provides access to the central veins
- Permits rapid infusion of medications or large amounts of fluids
- Allows clinicians to draw blood samples and measure central venous (CV) pressure
- Reduces the need for repeated venipunctures
- Reduces the risk of vein irritation

Drawbacks

- Increases the risk of life-threatening complications

Catheter types and uses

- Nontunneled: designed for short-term use
- Tunneled: designed for long-term use
- Peripherally inserted central catheters (PICCs): used when the patient requires infusions of caustic drugs or solutions
- Implanted port: used when an external catheter isn't suitable

Common CV insertion sites

- Subclavian vein
- Internal or external jugular vein
- Cephalic vein
- Basilic vein

Insertion site considerations

- Presence of scar tissue
- Possible interference with surgical site or other therapy
- Configuration of lung apices
- Patient's lifestyle and daily activities

Before insertion

- Explain the procedure to the patient.
- Place the patient in Trendelenburg's position.
- Prepare the insertion site: remove hair and clean the site with antiseptic solution.
- Assist with sterile drape application.
- Conscious sedation may be used; if so, the patient requires close observation.

During insertion

- Monitor patient tolerance.
- Assist as needed.
- Provide support to the patient.

After insertion

- Monitor for complications.
- Apply a transparent semipermeable dressing.
- Document the insertion.

Complications of CV therapy

- Pneumothorax, hemothorax, chylothorax, hydrothorax
- Air embolism
- Thrombus formation
- Perforation of vessel and adjacent organs
- Local infection
- Systemic infection

Complications of implanted port therapy

- Infection at injection site
- Skin breakdown
- Extravasation
- Thrombosis
- Fibrin sheath formation

Infusion maintenance

- Change the transparent semipermeable dressing whenever it becomes moist, loose, or soiled.
- Change the I.V. solution every 24 hours according to facility protocol.
- Change the I.V. tubing every 72 hours according to facility protocol.
- Flush the catheter with a two-way valve daily to every 8 hours (if not in use) or according to facility protocol.
- Change the gauze dressing at least every 48 hours.
- Change the intermittent injection caps at least every 7 days.

Port implantation and maintenance

- Explain the procedure to the patient and make sure he has signed a consent form.
- Monitor the patient during and after implantation for complications (infection, clotting, skin irritation).
- Change the dressing whenever its integrity is compromised.
- Change the needleless device or needle every 7 days.
- Flush every 4 weeks if not accessed.

What to document

- Status of the site
- Type of needle or port used
- Type of device used
- Procedure performed
- Patient's tolerance of the procedure
- Problems encountered and nursing interventions performed
- Type of dressing used
- Patient teaching performed and patient's understanding of teaching

■ Batter's box

CV therapy is used in several clinical situations. Fill in the blanks with the answer options below.

In CV therapy, _____ or _____ are infused directly into a major

                 1   2

vein. Commonly used during an _____ or when a patient's peripheral veins are

                                     3

inaccessible, CV therapy may also be used when a patient:

- needs _____ of a large volume of fluid

            4

- requires _____ infusions

            5

- requires _____ infusion therapy

            6

- needs infusion of _____ medications such as potassium

            7

- needs infusion of fluids with high _____ such as total parenteral nutrition

            8
  (TPN).

Options

A. drugs

B. emergency

C. fluids

D. infusion

E. irritating

F. long-term

G. multiple

H. osmolarity

> With CV therapy, you have direct access to a major route, leading straight back to little old me!

■ Strikeout

CV therapy offers many advantages over peripheral vein infusions. Of the following advantages, cross out those that don't apply to CV therapy.

1. Provides access to central veins

2. Allows for rapid infusion of medications or large amounts of fluids

3. Provides a way to draw arterial blood samples

4. Provides a way to measure CV pressure, an important indicator of circulatory function

5. Reduces need for repeated venipunctures, which decreases patient anxiety and preserves peripheral veins

6. Reduces risk of thrombus formation

7. Reduces risk of vein irritation from infusing irritating or caustic substances

8. Reduces risk of sepsis

Finish line

Identify the major vessels used in CV therapy shown in this illustration.

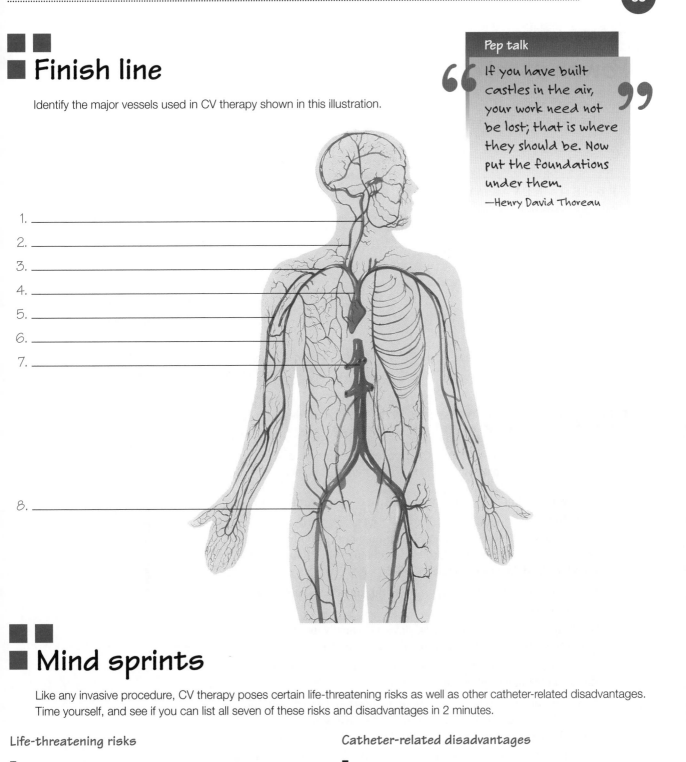

1. _____
2. _____
3. _____
4. _____
5. _____
6. _____
7. _____

8. _____

Mind sprints

Like any invasive procedure, CV therapy poses certain life-threatening risks as well as other catheter-related disadvantages. Time yourself, and see if you can list all seven of these risks and disadvantages in 2 minutes.

Life-threatening risks

- _____
- _____
- _____
- _____

Catheter-related disadvantages

- _____
- _____
- _____

Power stretch

Stretch your knowledge of CV circulation by first unscrambling the words on the left to reveal two major veins by which blood enters the right atrium. Then draw a line from the box to the specific veins that empty into it.

A. Right subclavian vein

B. Femoral vein

C. External jugular vein

D. Left brachiocephalic vein

E. Common iliac vein

F. Internal jugular vein

G. Left subclavian vein

H. Right brachiocephalic vein

I. Hepatic vein

RISPUREO   NEVA   AVCA

_ _ _ _ _ _ _ _   _ _ _ _   _ _ _ _

IREFOINR   NAVE   AAVC

_ _ _ _ _ _ _ _   _ _ _ _   _ _ _ _

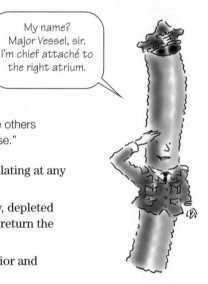

My name? Major Vessel, sir. I'm chief attaché to the right atrium.

Hit or miss

Some of the following statements about CV circulation are true, while others are false. Mark each statement with a "T" for "True" or an "F" for "False."

_____ 1. The average adult body contains about 10 L of blood circulating at any given time.

_____ 2. After delivering oxygen and nutrients throughout the body, depleted blood flows from capillaries into ever-widening veins that return the blood to the right side of the heart.

_____ 3. CV circulation enters the right ventricle through the superior and inferior venae cavae.

_____ 4. In CV therapy, the tip of the access device is usually inserted into either the superior vena cava or the inferior vena cava.

_____ 5. In the venae cavae, blood flows slowly around the tip of the access device, at about 500 ml/minute.

_____ 6. In a variation of CV therapy, a catheter is inserted through a peripheral vein and then passed all the way to the vena cava, sometimes threaded through two or more veins before reaching its final destination.

_____ 7. Usually, a CV access device is inserted into the subclavian vein or the internal jugular vein and then threaded through until it terminates in the inferior vena cava.

_____ 8. Because fluids are rapidly diluted by the venous circulation, highly concentrated or caustic fluids can be infused.

■ Match point

In CV therapy, an access device is inserted with its tip terminating in either the superior vena cava or the inferior vena cava. Match each commonly used CV pathway on the left with its corresponding description on the right.

1. _____

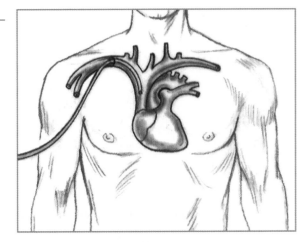

Description

A. Access device inserted peripherally into the basilic vein, terminating in the superior vena cava

B. Access device inserted into the internal jugular vein, terminating in superior vena cava

C. Access device inserted into the subclavian vein, terminating in superior vena cava

2. _____

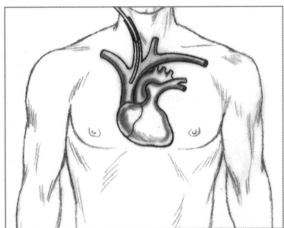

Although femoral veins in the legs are large vessels and feed into the inferior vena cava, they're typically used only when other sites aren't suitable because they carry an increased risk of complications.

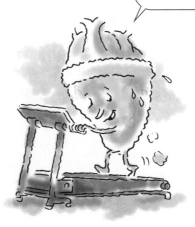

3. _____

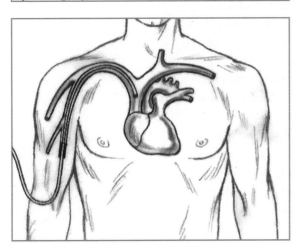

Jumble gym

Use these clues to help you unscramble the four different types of catheters used in CV therapy. Then use the circled letters to answer this question:

Question: To ease the insertion and placement of CV access devices, many newer models come in variable lengths, with smaller lumens and longer what?

1. Usually designed for short-term use, such as brief continuation of I.V. therapy following hospitalization; not appropriate for patients starting long-term I.V. therapy

N E D N U L E N O N T   H E R E C A T T

— ◯ — — — ◯ — — — —   — — — ◯ — — —

2. Cuffed and usually made of silicone; better suited for home care patients requiring long-term use

L U T E D E N N   C S S E A C   D V I E C E

— ◯ — — — — ◯ —   — — — — ◯ —   — — — — — —

3. Long-armed or long-lined and one of the most commonly used types; generally used for infusion of caustic drugs or solutions

L E A R Y P H I P L E R   D E S I N R E T   E L T R C A N
H E A R T C E T

— — ◯ — — — — — — — —   — — — — — — — — —   — — — ◯ — —

◯ — — — — — —

4. Functions like a long-term catheter; used when an external catheter isn't suitable

T I N P E L M A D   S R O P T

◯ — — — — — — — —   — — ◯ —

Answer: __ __ __ __ __ __ __ __ __ __ __

> ### Pep talk
>
> " Circumstances may cause interruptions and delays, but never lose sight of your goal. Prepare yourself in every way you can by increasing your knowledge and adding to your experience, so that you can make the most of opportunity when it occurs. "
>
> —Mario Andretti

■ ■
■ You make the call

Identify the type of access device shown in the illustration, and briefly explain how it's inserted.

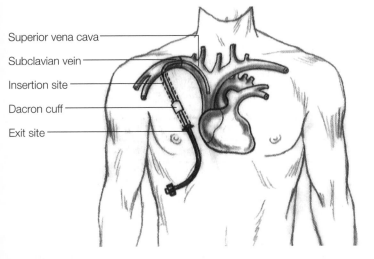

Superior vena cava

Subclavian vein

Insertion site

Dacron cuff

Exit site

Catheter type: _____

How it's inserted: _____

_____

_____

_____

_____

_____

_____

■ ■
■ Strikeout

These statements pertain to tunneled and nontunneled CV access devices. Cross out all of the incorrect statements.

1. Tunneled and nontunneled access devices are radiopaque, so their placement can be checked by X-ray.

2. The silicone used in tunneled access devices is less physiologically compatible than polyurethane or polyvinyl and, therefore, is more likely to cause thrombosis and irritation or damage to the vein lining.

3. Nontunneled access devices directly access the subclavian vein.

4. A tunneled CV access device has a cuff that encourages tissue growth within the tunnel.

5. Within 1 week to 10 days after placement of a tunneled access device, new tissue growth anchors the access device in place and keeps bacteria out of the venous circulation.

6. Most cuffs used in tunneled access devices contain silver ions that provide antibacterial protection for about 3 months.

7. Nontunneled access devices are changed every 5 days to prevent infection.

8. Tunneled access devices are used in patients who have poor peripheral venous access or who need long-term daily infusions.

Do you know which patients are prime candidates for tunneled access devices?

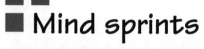

Mind sprints

Identify four medications that are given by tunneled CV access device and at least six conditions that require this type of infusion. Time yourself, and see how many you can list in 2 minutes.

Medications

- _____
- _____
- _____
- _____

Conditions

- _____
- _____
- _____
- _____
- _____
- _____

Boxing match

Use all of the syllables in the boxes shown to fill in the answers to clues about the names of some commonly used CV access devices. The number of syllables for each answer is shown in parentheses.

A C	BRO	GRO	HICK	LINE	LONG	~~LU~~
MAN	~~MEN~~	~~MUL~~	SHONG	~~TI~~	VI	

1. Short-term access device with double, triple, or quadruple lumen at ¾″ (1.9 cm) intervals; allows infusion of multiple solutions through the same catheter (4) M U L T I L U M E N

2. Long-term tunneled access device used for patients with a heparin allergy; has closed end with pressure-sensitive two-way valve and single or double lumen (2) _ _ _ _ _ _ _ _

3. Open-ended, long-term tunneled access device with a clamp; has a Dacron cuff 11¾″ (29.9 cm) from the hub (2) _ _ _ _ _ _ _

4. Single, small-lumen tunneled access device designed for long-term use; commonly used in children and elderly patients (3) _ _ _ _ _ _ _

5. Peripherally inserted long-term catheter; has single or double lumen (2) _ _ _ _ _ – _ _ _ _

■ Batter's box

Use the options below to complete these statements about PICCs.

Also known as *long-arm* or *long-line catheters*, PICCs are inserted through a

_____ vein, with the tip ending in the _____ . If the catheter
₁ ₂

tip is located outside the vena cava, it's no longer considered a _____
₃

catheter and should be removed.

Generally, PICCs are used in patients needing _____ or infusions of
₄

_____ drugs or solutions. They're especially useful when the patient doesn't
₅

have a reliable route for _____ I.V. therapy. A PICC may also be ordered
₆

when a patient has a chest injury due to _____ or _____ or
₇ ₈

_____ problems due to chronic obstructive pulmonary disease.
₉

Using a peripheral insertion site for CV access helps prevent problems such as

_____ that may occur with a CV access device that's inserted into the chest.
₁₀

Options
A. burns
B. caustic
C. central
D. peripheral
E. pneumothorax
F. respiratory
G. short-term
H. transfusions
I. trauma
J. vena cava

■ Gear up!

In case your facility doesn't use a preassembled disposable tray for CV access device insertion, you'll need to know which equipment to gather before this procedure. Check off all the equipment that you'll need.

☐ CV access device
☐ Extra syringes and blood sample containers (for venous samples, if ordered)
☐ Heparin or saline flush solution
☐ Implantable pump
☐ Infusion pump
☐ Linen-saver pad
☐ Local anesthetic
☐ 3-ml syringe with 25G needle (for introduction of anesthetic)

☐ Antimicrobial solution
☐ Scissors
☐ Sterile dressing
☐ Sterile gauze pads
☐ Sterile mask, gown, and gloves
☐ Sterile syringe (for blood samples)
☐ Sterile towels or drapes
☐ Suture material
☐ Tuberculin syringe
☐ Implanted port
☐ Warming blanket

Remember, equipment is important!

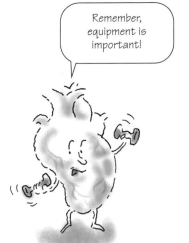

Hit or miss

Some of these statements about PICC devices are true; others are false. Mark the true statements with a "T" and the false ones with an "F."

_____ 1. All PICCs include a built-in guide wire to ease advancement through the vein.

_____ 2. To infuse blood or blood products through a PICC, you should use a catheter that's 18G or larger.

_____ 3. Tuberculin syringes are preferred when administering medications through a PICC.

_____ 4. Only doctors can insert tunneled access devices and PICCs in patients because these devices require surgery.

_____ 5. One type of PICC—an extended peripheral catheter—is inserted through the axillary vein and terminates in the inferior vena cava.

_____ 6. Some PICCs have antithrombogenic properties that minimize the risk of blood clots and phlebitis.

_____ 7. PICCs are a good alternative and often a last resort for patients with bruises, scarring, or sclerosis of the veins.

_____ 8. Bedside ultrasound can be helpful in assessing vein suitability when using a PICC.

_____ 9. PICCs usually range from 14G to 24G in diameter and from $7\frac{3}{4}''$ to $23\frac{1}{2}''$ (19.5 to 59.5 cm) in length.

_____ 10. Because PICCs are made of silicone rubber they don't require frequent monitoring for signs of phlebitis and thrombus formation.

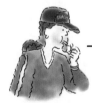

Coaching session

Guidelines for using CV access devices

When using a CV access device, keep these general guidelines in mind:
• Know the gauge and purpose of each lumen.
• Use the same lumen for the same task; label lumens, as necessary, to prevent confusion.
• Apply dressings after insertion.
• Handle the catheter gently.
• Observe frequently for kinks, tears, or leaks.
• Flush the catheter to clear the line and prevent occlusion (follow facility protocol).
• Assess frequently for signs of infection and clot formation.

Finish line

The Arrow catheter, a commonly used peripherally inserted long-line catheter, includes an introducer needle, slide clamp, needle-free injection cap, and peel-away contamination guard, as well as staggered infusion ports and catheter anchoring devices. Identify these features on this illustration.

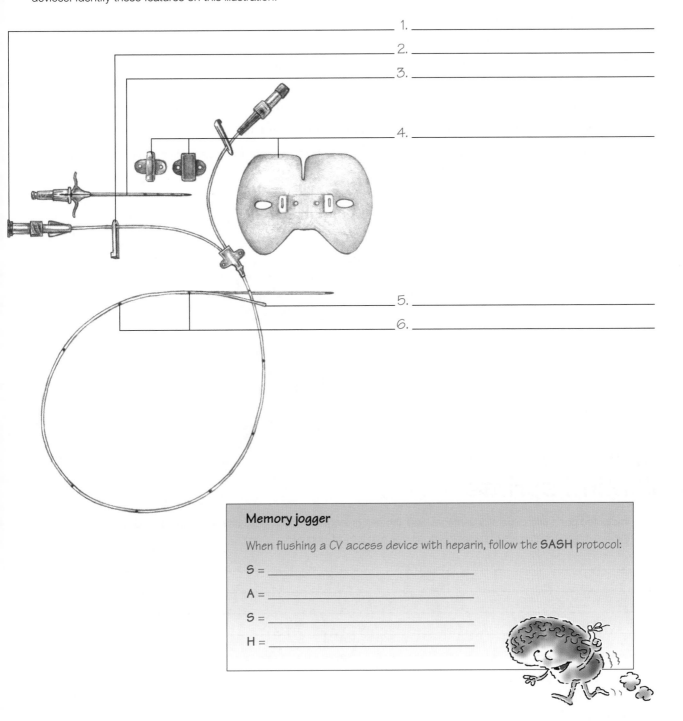

1. _____

2. _____

3. _____

4. _____

5. _____

6. _____

Memory jogger

When flushing a CV access device with heparin, follow the **SASH** protocol:

S = _____

A = _____

S = _____

H = _____

■ Strikeout

The following statements pertain to implanted ports. Cross out all of the incorrect statements.

1. An implanted port functions like a long-term access device except that it doesn't have any external parts.

2. An implanted port is inserted in a pocket under the patient's skin.

3. The indwelling catheter that's attached to the port is surgically tunneled until the catheter tip lies in the vena cava.

4. The implanted port is commonly threaded through either the femoral vein at the shoulder or the common ileal vein at the base of the neck.

5. An implanted port is also suitable for epidural, intra-arterial, or intraperitoneal placement.

6. Using an implanted port for self-infusion of medication is comfortable and extremely convenient for the patient.

7. An implanted port is typically used for infusion therapy lasting 6 months or longer, whereas an implantable pump is used for continuous low-volume infusions.

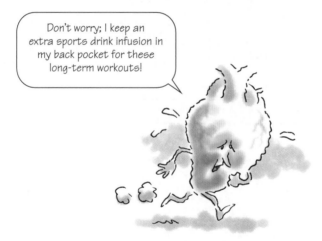

Don't worry; I keep an extra sports drink infusion in my back pocket for these long-term workouts!

■ Mind sprints

Implanted ports offer several advantages over the use of long-term CV access devices. See how many of the five major advantages of implanted ports you can list in 1 minute.

- _____
- _____
- _____
- _____
- _____

■ Batter's box

Complete the information about implantable pumps by filling in the blanks with the appropriate words from the options. Use each option only once.

An implantable pump is usually placed in a _____ pocket made in the

1

abdomen below the _____ . An implantable pump has two chambers

2

separated by a _____ . One chamber contains the I.V. solution, and the

3

other contains a _____ . The charging fluid chamber exerts continuous

4

pressure on the bellows, forcing the infusion through the _____ catheter

5

into a central vein. The pump also has an auxiliary _____ that can be

6

used to deliver bolus injections of medication. Generally, the pump is indicated for

patients who require continuous _____ infusions.

7

Options

A. bellows

B. charging fluid

C. low-volume

D. septum

E. silicone outlet

F. subcutaneous

G. umbilicus

■ Finish line

Label the parts of the implantable pump shown here.

Pep talk

Change is the law of life. And those who look only to the past or present are certain to miss the future.
—John F. Kennedy

Top view

Cross-sectional view

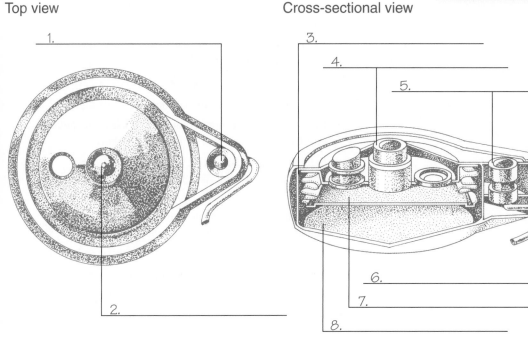

1. _____

2. _____

3. _____

4. _____

5. _____

6. _____

7. _____

8. _____

■ Mind sprints

With the exception of PICC insertions, CV access devices are usually inserted by a doctor. Unless it's an emergency procedure, the insertion site will vary and the patient may even collaborate in selecting a site. See if you can list, in 2 minutes or less, seven factors that affect insertion site selection.

■ _____

■ _____

■ _____

■ _____

■ _____

■ _____

■ _____

■ Power stretch

Stretch your knowledge of CV insertion sites by first unscrambling the words on the left to reveal five of the most commonly used veins. Then draw a line from each vein to its descriptions on the right.

RATENLIN
GRULAJU

— — — — — — — —
— — — — — — —

LIBCAIS

— — — — — — —

LIVBUSANCA

— — — — — — — — — —

ERXATELN RAGULUJ

— — — — — — — —
— — — — — — —

HIPELCAC

— — — — — — — —

A. Provides easy access and a short, direct route to the superior vena cava and CV circulation

B. Is commonly used in children, but not infants

C. Has the least risk of major complications

D. Shouldn't be used to administer highly caustic medications

E. Right side provides a more direct route to the vena cava than the left side

F. Is located proximal to the angle of Louis

G. Is often preferred because it's large and straight

H. Is a large vein; has high volume of blood flow, making clot formation and vein irritation less likely

I. Is located at a sharp angle below the shoulder, sometimes making it difficult to thread an access device through it

J. Is located proximal to the carotid artery, which can sometimes lead to serious complications

K. Makes it sometimes difficult to keep dressing in place

L. Makes it easier to keep dressing in place

M. Allows greatest patient mobility after insertion

N. Is often tortuous, especially in elderly patients

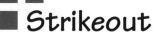

Strikeout

The femoral vein may be used for CV therapy when other sites aren't suitable. Cross out the incorrect statements about the femoral vein.

1. Although the femoral veins are large veins, using them for access device insertion entails some complications.

2. Insertion of an access device in the femoral vein is usually less difficult in a larger patient.

3. Insertion of an access device in a femoral vein may result in puncture of the local lymph nodes.

4. The femoral vein site inherently carries a lower risk of local infection than other veins.

5. When a femoral vein is used in CV therapy, the patient's leg needs to be kept straight; however, movement isn't generally limited.

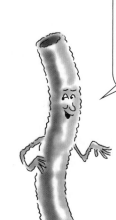

I don't mind getting picked last for the team. The way I look at it, being a femoral vein, I end up with fewer holes and have less chance of getting blamed when things go wrong!

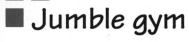

Jumble gym

Use the clues to help you unscramble words representing serious complications that can occur with use of the internal jugular vein for CV therapy. Then use the circled letters to answer the question posed.

Question: A patient who suffers all of these complications can end up with irreversible what?

1. Can result because of its close proximity to the internal jugular vein

P U C E T R U N D   R A I D C O T   Y E A R R T

_ _ _ _ _ _ ◯ _   _ ◯ _ _ _ _   ◯ _ _ _ _

2. Can get out of hand quickly once it begins

O L D N U T C L O N E R   H R A E H M O G E R

_ _ _ _ ◯ _ _ _ _ _   _ _ _ _ ◯ _ _ ◯◯ _

3. Can occur if air gets in the vein

B L I M O E   _ _ ◯ _ _ ◯

4. Can result when the vein becomes occluded

D E P I M E D   O L D B O   W L O F

_ ◯ _ _ _ _ _   _ _ _ _ ◯   _ _ _ _

Answer: _ _ _ _ _   _ _ _ _ _ _

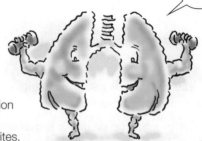

Have I met Catheter Tip yet? Well, I've seen her at several procedures, but we've never been formally introduced.

Cross-training

Proximity to certain bones, organs, vessels, and other anatomical landmarks can make CV access device insertion difficult and sometimes risky. Complete the following crossword puzzle to test your knowledge of these body sites.

Across

2. Proximity to this area increases the risk of infection when a femoral vein is used.

5. The practitioner aims under the clavicle for this area when inserting an access device into the subclavian vein (three words).

6. Also called the *collarbone*, this landmark is used in subclavian insertion.

7. Recent surgery at this site may preclude use of the internal and external jugular veins.

8. These may become punctured with insertion of a CV access device into the femoral vein (two words).

9. The subclavian site is in close proximity to this region's major vessels.

Down

1. This space at the bend of the elbow is the site of peripheral insertions (two words).

3. Venipuncture of the subclavian vein is close to the apex of this organ.

4. This artery is proximal to the internal jugular vein.

Mind sprints

There are four notable concerns to keep in mind when you select a site for insertion of a CV access device. See if you can identify all four of them in 2 minutes or less.

■ _____

■ _____

■ _____

■ _____

■ Hit or miss

Preparing the patient for CV therapy includes providing him with accurate and thorough patient teaching. Mark each of these patient-teaching statements with a "T" for "True" or an "F" for "False."

_____ 1. "Bedside CV insertion is a sterile procedure, so expect the practitioner and nurses to be wearing gowns, masks, and gloves; you may need to wear a mask, too."

_____ 2. "In order to access the subclavian or jugular vein, you'll need to be placed flat on your back with your feet dangling over the bed."

_____ 3. "You can expect to feel a stinging sensation from the local anesthetic and a little bit of pressure during access device insertion."

_____ 4. "This is so routine that you won't require any other tests before or after the procedure."

■ Batter's box

Fill in the blanks with answer options that complete the following patient-teaching information about CV access device insertion.

The primary responsibility for explaining the procedure and its goals rests with

the _____ . Your role may include allaying the patient's
           1

_____ and answering any questions about _____
        2   3

restrictions, _____ concerns, and management regimens.
                      4

In explaining self-care measures, be sure to teach the patient how to perform

_____ , and have him demonstrate it to you at least twice. This is
        5

especially important in preventing _____ . Also teach him how to
                                              6

change the _____ and how to _____ the device.
                    7   8

Options
A. air embolism
B. cosmetic
C. practitioner
D. dressing
E. flush
F. fears
G. movement
H. Valsalva's maneuver

Pep talk

66 You must see your goals clearly and specifically before you can set out for them. Hold them in your mind until they become second nature. 99

—Les Brown

■ Starting lineup

Put the following steps in the correct order to show how you would set up equipment for insertion of a CV access device at the patient's bedside.

Prime and calibrate any pressure monitoring setups.

Attach the tubing to the solution container.

Cover all open ends of the access device with sealed caps.

Fill the syringes with saline or heparin flush solutions, based on facility policy and procedure.

Recheck all connections to make sure they're secure.

Prime the tubing with the solution.

■ You make the call

Identify the patient position illustrated below, and briefly explain why it's used in CV access device insertion

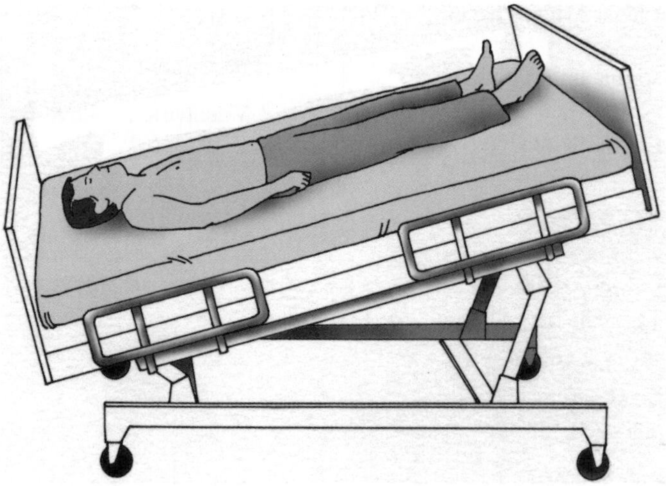

Position: _____

Why it's used: _____

_____

_____

_____

_____

_____

_____

_____

■ Batter's box

Complete the following information about preparing the patient for CV access device insertion using answers from the options below.

Although specific steps may vary, the same basic procedure is used whether access

device insertion is done at the bedside or in the _____ . Before the

practitioner inserts the access device, you need to _____ the patient and
                                                              2

prepare the _____ . Some patients require _____ for the
                  3   4

access device to be placed, and they must be carefully monitored by staff trained in the

procedure.

   Place the patient in _____ position. If the _____ vein is
                              5   6

to be used, place a rolled towel or blanket between the patient's _____ .
                                                                          7

Doing so allows for more direct access and may prevent puncture of the

_____ or adjacent vessels. If the _____ vein is to be used,
        8   9

place a rolled blanket under the opposite shoulder to extend the _____
                                                                          10

and make anatomical landmarks more visible.

> **Options**
> A. insertion site
> B. internal jugular
> C. lung apex
> D. neck
> E. operating room
> F. position
> G. scapulae
> H. sedation
> I. subclavian
> J. Trendelenburg's

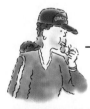

Coaching session
Hair removal before CV access device insertion

The Infusion Nurses Society and other infection-control practitioners recommend clipping the hair close to the skin rather than shaving it before CV access device insertion.

Saved from a close shave
Shaving can cause site irritation and create multiple small, open wounds on the skin, increasing the risk of infection. To avoid irritation, clip the patient's hair with single-use clipper blades.

Don't forget to rinse
After removing the patient's hair, rinse the skin with saline solution to remove any hair clippings. You may also wash the skin with soap and water before the actual skin prep to remove surface dirt and body oils.

■ Starting lineup

Put these steps in the correct sequence to show how you would prepare a site for CV access device insertion.

Clip the patient's hair from around the site to prevent infection from microorganisms, as needed.	
Place a linen-saver pad under the site to prevent soiling.	
Adjust sterile drapes to uncover the patient's eyes, if necessary.	
Swab the site with chlorhexidine using a back-and-forth motion.	

■ Strikeout

Nurses have several important responsibilities during and immediately after the CV access device insertion procedure. Cross out the incorrect statements regarding this procedure.

1. During the procedure, the nurse is responsible for monitoring the patient and providing emotional support.

2. The practitioner, not the nurse, usually prepares the equipment, including opening the CV access kit, which requires aseptic technique.

3. In many cases, the nurse is asked to perform fluoroscopy and inject contrast dye to assist with access device placement.

4. After the access device is inserted, the nurse may need to obtain several venous blood samples.

5. Typically, the nurse collects blood samples by using a sterile 10-ml syringe or by accessing a saline lock at the end of the port with a Vacutainer.

6. Whenever the access device hub is open to air, such as when changing syringes during blood sampling, the nurse must tell the patient to take a deep breath.

7. After the insertion process, the nurse applies a dressing to the site and documents the procedure.

8. It's especially important for the nurse to monitor the patient's cardiac and respiratory status during and after access device insertion to detect complications.

9. Elevating the head of the patient's bed 45 degrees after applying the dressing will ensure that the infusion flows by gravity.

Match point

Monitoring the patient involves checking for signs and symptoms of complications related to the CV access device's placement during insertion. Match the likely complication on the left with the signs and symptoms on the right.

Likely complication

1. Air embolism _____
2. Punctured lung _____
3. Misplaced access device in right atrium or right ventricle _____

Signs and symptoms

A. Arrhythmias

B. Dyspnea, shortness of breath, sudden chest pain

C. Respiratory distress, unequal breath sounds, decreased blood pressure, increased CV pressure

Memory jogger

When changing caps on the central venous access device, think of the three Cs:

C _____

C _____

C _____

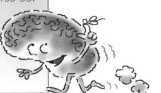

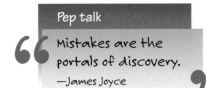

Pep talk

Mistakes are the portals of discovery.

—James Joyce

Mind sprints

Think fast! In 1 minute or less, list three possible problems that can result from a poorly placed access device, especially one inserted into the internal or external jugular vein.

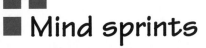

- _____
- _____
- _____

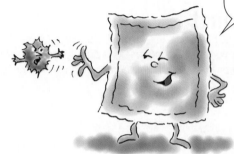

Remember to keep the access device site clean and dry, and keep me occlusive to prevent contamination.

Starting lineup

Put these steps in the correct sequence to show how you would apply a sterile dressing over the insertion site of a short-term catheter or the exit site of a PICC or tunneled access device.

Cover the site with a transparent semipermeable dressing.	
Label the dressing with the date and time, your initials, and the catheter length.	
Clean the site with chlorhexidine using the same method as the initial skin preparation.	
Seal the dressing with nonporous tape, checking that all edges are well secured.	

Mind sprints

What five pieces of information are essential to document in the nurse's notes or I.V. flow sheet following insertion of a CV access device? See how many you can list in 2 minutes.

- _____
- _____
- _____
- _____
- _____

■ Batter's box

Fill in the missing words using the answer options below to complete these statements about routine care measures needed to maintain CV infusions.

Maintaining CV infusions includes providing _____ care of the CV

(1)

access device insertion site and of the access device and _____ .

(2)

Also expect to:

- change the transparent _____ dressing whenever it becomes

(3)

_____ , loose, or soiled

(4)

- change the I.V. tubing and _____

(5)

- _____ the access device

(6)

- change the access device _____

(7)

- administer a _____ or obtain _____ , if needed

(8) (9)

- record your _____ findings and _____ according

(10) (11)

to facility policy.

> **Options**
> A. assessment
> B. blood samples
> C. cap
> D. flush
> E. interventions
> F. meticulous
> G. moist
> H. secondary infusion
> I. semipermeable
> J. solution
> K. tubing

■ Gear up!

Many facilities use a preassembled dressing tray that contains all the equipment needed for a routine dressing change. Check off the items that should be included.

- ☐ Chlorhexidine swabs
- ☐ Clean gloves
- ☐ Irrigation solution
- ☐ Local anesthetic for injection
- ☐ Sterile drape
- ☐ Sterile gloves and masks
- ☐ Sutures
- ☐ Syringe
- ☐ Transparent semipermeable dressing

> Keep up the pace. You're doing a great job!

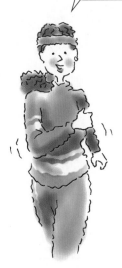

■ In the ballpark

Your patient's CV access device dressing, solution, tubing, and intermittent injection caps must be changed regularly, following strict aseptic technique and facility policy, to prevent infection. Circle the correct number to indicate how often each should be changed.

Dressing	Every 8 hours	Every 24 hours	Every 4 to 7 days
Solution	Every 4 hours	Every 24 hours	Every 48 hours
Tubing	Every 8 hours	Every 48 hours	Every 72 hours
Caps	Every 12 hours	Every 24 hours	Every 7 days

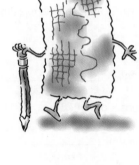

Don't forget to document all dressing, solution, and tubing changes in your nurse's notes and on the I.V. flowchart, if your facility uses one

Pep talk

" Knowing is not enough; we must apply. Willing is not enough; we must do. "
—Johann Wolfgang von Goethe

■ Photo finish

Identify and briefly explain each step of changing a CV access device dressing.

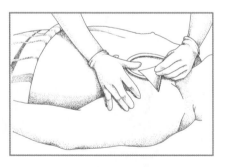

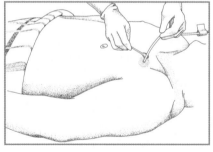

1. _____

2. _____

3. _____

Mind sprints

Here's an easy one. List four signs of infiltration or infection you may see when examining the CV access device insertion site during a CV dressing change. See if you can list them all in less than 1 minute.

- _____
- _____
- _____
- _____

Starting lineup

Now put these statements in correct order to show how you would change a CV dressing.

Put on clean gloves and remove the old dressing.	
Check the position of the access device and the insertion site for infiltration or infection.	
Wash your hands, and then place the patient in a comfortable position.	
Put on sterile gloves, and clean the skin around the access device with chlorhexidine using a back-and-forth or side-to-side motion.	
Prepare a sterile field. Open the bag, placing it away from the sterile field, but within reach.	
Redress the site with a transparent semipermeable dressing.	
Discard all used items properly, then reposition the patient comfortably.	
Inspect the old dressing for signs of infection. Culture discharge at the site or on the old dressing (if needed), and dispose of the old dressing and gloves in the bag	
Label the dressing with the date, time, and your initials.	

■ Hit or miss

Mark each of these statements about maintaining CV access devices with a "T" for "True" or an "F" for "False."

_____ 1. You should wear a mask and gloves whenever you change a patient's CV solution or tubing.

_____ 2. You should always change the solution and tubing at the same time.

_____ 3. To eliminate the need for having the patient perform Valsalva's maneuver each time the access device hub is open to air, many facilities use a connecting tubing between the access device hub and I.V. tubing that allows the tubing to be clamped during changes.

_____ 4. CV access devices are routinely flushed with saline solution at least once per day.

_____ 5. If a heparinized saline flush solution is used, you should always administer the highest possible heparin concentration.

_____ 6. The frequency of flushing depends on the type of access device and the facility's policy; no flushing is needed with a continuous infusion through a single-lumen access device.

_____ 7. Obtaining a blood return of 3 to 5 ml of free-flowing blood is recommended before use of the access device.

_____ 8. Flushing an access device with heparin or normal saline solution before and after the administration of incompatible medications is recommended.

_____ 9. You should always use clean technique when changing access device caps.

_____ 10. Secondary infusions are commonly piggybacked into a side port or Y-port of a primary infusion.

■ Strikeout

Cross out any incorrect statements within this set of step-by-step instructions for safely drawing blood from a CV access device.

Step 1: To draw blood using an evacuated tube, first wash your hands and put on sterile gloves.

Step 2: Then stop the I.V. infusion and place an injection cap on the lumen of the access device.

Step 3: If multiple infusions are running, wait until only one infusion is left running before stopping the infusion to collect the blood sample.

Step 4: Clean the end of the injection cap with heparin solution.

Step 5: Place a 5-ml lavender-top evacuated tube into its plastic sleeve, and use this tube to collect and discard the filling volume of the access device, plus an extra 5 to 10 ml of blood.

Step 6: Insert the needleless device into the injection cap; then, when blood stops flowing into the tube, remove and discard the tube following facility policy.

Step 7: After you've collected the ordered blood samples in the appropriate evacuated tubes, flush the access device with saline solution using a 10-ml syringe, and resume the infusion; if you're not going to use the lumen immediately, heparinize the access device.

Step 8: Failure to get blood to flow from the access device using the above technique means that the access device is completely occluded; the only alternative is to use a syringe to obtain the blood sample.

■■ ■ Power stretch

Stretch your knowledge of maintaining CV therapy by first unscrambling the words on the left to reveal four common infusion-related problems. Then draw a line from each of these problems to the ways it's usually detected or corrected.

KINDEK
AESCCS IEVEDC

_ _ _ _ _ _

_ _ _ _ _ _   _ _ _ _ _ _

IFRNIB HASTEH

_ _ _ _ _ _   _ _ _ _ _ _

CETDNOCENSDI
CSCSEA DVEEIC

_ _ _ _ _ _ _ _ _ _ _ _

_ _ _ _ _ _   _ _ _ _ _ _

SCECSA ICVDEE
RATE

_ _ _ _ _ _   _ _ _ _ _ _

_ _ _ _

A. May be surgically removed

B. Can be fixed by clamping the access device and changing the I.V. extension set

C. Can be corrected under guided fluoroscopy using aseptic technique

D. Can be dissolved by instilling a thrombolytic agent

E. Detected by X-rays

F. Can result in blood backup, fluid leak, or air embolism

G. Can be corrected with proper taping and positioning

H. Makes withdrawing blood or infusing fluid difficult

I. Can be caused by patient movement or a loose connection to the tubing

J. Can be prevented by using nonserrated clamps

K. If ultimately broken, entire CV line can be replaced

■■ ■ Match point

Complications can occur at any time during CV therapy. Match each complication on the left with its description on the right.

Complication

1. Collapsed lung _____

2. Arterial puncture _____

3. Sepsis _____

Description

A. The most common complication of access device insertion; may be minimal or a medical emergency

B. The most serious systemic complication; can lead to death

C. The second most common life-threatening complication; can lead to hypovolemic shock

Monitoring for CV-related complications is a workout in itself! Remember to always keep on your toes, and react quickly to any sign of a problem.

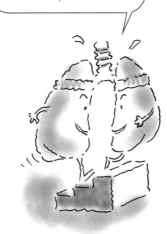

Cross-training

Fill in the clues of this crossword puzzle to uncover the risks of CV therapy.

Across

2. An abnormal connection between the brachiocephalic vein and the subclavian artery and caused by perforation by guide wire on insertion into blood vessel

5. A collapsed lung from puncture during access device insertion

6. A lymph node puncture that leaks lymph fluid into the pleural cavity

9. A serious infection often resulting from *Staphylococcus* or *Candida* infections (two words)

10. A clot that forms in a blood vessel

Down

1. Intake of air into CV system during access device insertion or tubing changes (two words)

3. Contamination confined to the access device insertion site and caused by failure to maintain aseptic technique or problems with the dressing (two words)

4. A large blood vessel puncture with bleeding inside or outside lung

7. An infusion of solution into the chest cavity through a perforated access device

8. A systemic infection caused by contamination or failure to maintain aseptic technique

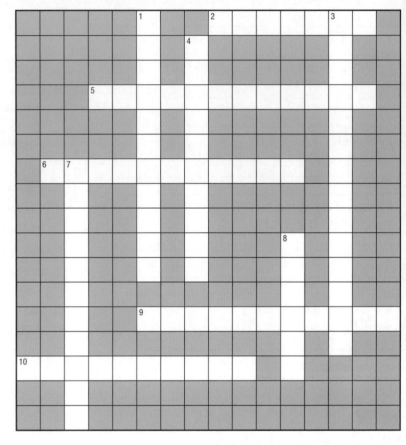

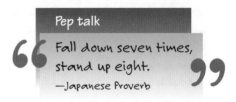

Pep talk

" Fall down seven times, stand up eight.
—Japanese Proverb "

> I must have blown a lung with that last access device insertion!

Mind sprints

Quickly list four symptoms that you might detect in a patient who has suffered a severe pneumothorax as a result of insertion of CV access device insertion.

- _____
- _____
- _____
- _____

Memory jogger

If unchecked, pneumothorax may progress to tension pneumothorax, a medical emergency. To remember the signs and symptoms of tension pneumothorax, remember that you have to **ACT** fast to protect your patient:

A _____

C _____

T _____

Match point

Show that you can recognize the complications associated with CV therapy by matching each set of signs and symptoms on the left with the complication it describes on the right.

Signs and symptoms

1. Redness, warmth, tenderness, and swelling at insertion site; possible exudate; local rash or pustules; fever, chills, and malaise _____

2. Respiratory distress, unequal breath sounds, weak pulse, increased CV pressure, decreased blood pressure, churning murmur over precordium, change in or loss of consciousness _____

3. Fever and chills without other apparent reason, leukocytosis, nausea and vomiting, malaise, elevated urine glucose level _____

4. Edema at puncture site; ipsilateral swelling of arm, neck, and face; pain; fever and malaise; tachycardia _____

5. Chest pain, dyspnea, cyanosis, decreased breath sounds on affected side, abnormal chest X-ray _____

Complication

A. Air embolism

B. Local infection

C. Pneumothorax

D. Systemic infection

E. Thrombosis

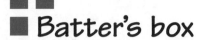

Batter's box

Complete this information about PICC-specific complications by filling in the blanks with answers from the options.

The most common PICC complication is _____ , or painful

_____ of a vein. Typically occurring during the first 72 hours, it's more

common in _____ insertions and when a _____ catheter

is used. Some patients develop _____ phlebitis; however, this usually

occurs later in therapy. Other complications that occur with traditional CV lines,

such as _____ and _____ , tend to occur rarely with

PICC therapy because the catheter insertion site is _____ and below

the level of the _____ .

Expect a minimal amount of _____ from the PICC site for the first

24 hours, during which time a _____ should be kept in place.

Options
A. air embolism
B. bacterial
C. bleeding
D. heart
E. inflammation
F. large-gauge
G. left-sided
H. peripheral
I. pneumothorax
J. pressure dressing
K. mechanical phlebitis

Match point

Knowing what to do when complications arise is critical to your practice. Match the complication on the left with its nursing interventions on the right.

Complication

1. Thrombosis _____
2. Pneumothorax _____
3. Air embolism _____
4. Local infection _____
5. Phlebitis _____
6. Sepsis _____

Nursing interventions

A. Monitor temperature frequently; culture the site; redress aseptically; administer antibiotics or antifungals as ordered; remove the access device if ordered.

B. Notify the practitioner; infuse thrombolytic agent as ordered; verify through diagnostic studies; avoid using the affected limb for subsequent venipunctures.

C. Stop the infusion and notify the practitioner; remove the access device or assist with removal; administer oxygen as ordered; set up and assist with chest tube insertion.

D. Draw central and peripheral blood cultures; if cultures match or are positive, remove the access device and culture the tip, as ordered; administer antibiotics as ordered; assess for other sources of infection; monitor vital signs closely.

E. Apply warm, moist compresses to the upper arm; elevate the affected extremity; restrict activity to mild exercise; notify the practitioner if drainage occurs at insertion site or temperature increases; remove the access device if ordered.

F. Clamp the access device immediately; cover the catheter exit site; turn the patient onto his left side with his head down; instruct the patient to avoid Valsalva's maneuver; administer oxygen; notify the practitioner.

■■ ■ Strikeout

Cross out any incorrect statements within this step-by-step description of CV access device removal.

Step 1: Check the patient's record or other documentation for the most recent placement confirmed by X-ray to trace the access device's path as it exits the body.

Step 2: Make sure backup assistance is available in case complications develop during removal.

Step 3: Explain the procedure to the patient, and tell him that he'll be instructed to take a deep breath as the access device is withdrawn.

Step 4: Gather all of the necessary equipment.

Step 5: Position the patient sitting upright on the edge of the bed.

Step 6: Wash your hands and put on clean gloves.

Step 7: Stop infusing all medications, but maintain a saline infusion to keep the vein open.

Step 8: Remove the old dressing.

Step 9: Inspect the site for signs of drainage or inflammation.

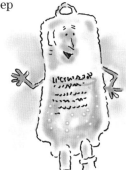

Well, all good things must come to an end—even a long-term CV infusion.

■■ ■ Starting lineup

Now show that you know the actual CV access device removal procedure by putting these steps in their proper order.

Inspect the access device to see if any pieces broke off during the removal. If so, notify the practitioner immediately and monitor the patient closely for signs of distress.	
Place a transparent semipermeable dressing over the site, and label the dressing with the date and time of removal and your initials.	
Properly dispose of the I.V. tubing and equipment you used.	
Clip the sutures and remove the access device in a slow, even motion as the patient performs Valsalva's maneuver.	
Continue to monitor the patient and the insertion site frequently for the next few hours for evidence of air emboli and insidious bleeding.	
Apply antimicrobial or antibiotic ointment to the insertion site to seal it.	

■ Hit or miss

Mark each statement regarding port implantation and infusion with a "T" for "True" and an "F" for "False."

_____ 1. An implanted port consists of a silicone catheter attached to a titanium, stainless steel, or plastic reservoir covered by a self-sealing silicone rubber septum.

_____ 2. The implanted port is surgically implanted under the skin in the patient's neck.

_____ 3. An implanted port may be used for intermittent delivery of chemotherapy, I.V. fluids, pain control, medications, and blood products; it's also sometimes used to administer TPN solutions.

_____ 4. Use of an intermittent infusion device or lock with an implanted port tends to increase the number of venipunctures, so such devices aren't commonly used.

_____ 5. There are two basic types of implanted ports: top entry and side entry.

_____ 6. The type of port selected depends primarily on the type of therapy needed and how often the port must be accessed.

_____ 7. To avoid damaging the port's silicone rubber septum, only straight, conventional needles are used with an implanted port.

■ You make the call

Identify the type of implanted port used in the illustration, and briefly explain how it's accessed.

Septum

Silicone catheter

Type of VAP: _____

How it's accessed: _____

_____

_____

_____

Pep talk

> You can have anything you want if you want it desperately enough. You must want it with an exuberance that erupts through the skin and joins the energy that created the world.
>
> —Sheila Graham

■ ■
■ Three-point conversion

Unlike a conventional hypodermic needle, a noncoring needle has a deflected point, which slices the septum of an implanted port instead of coring it. Identify the needle or set shown in each of these illustrations and briefly explain why it's used.

1.
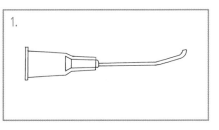

2.
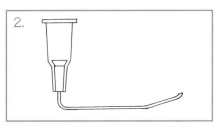

3.
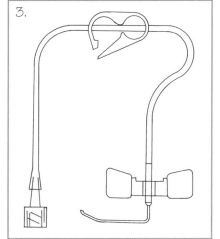

1. _____
_____

2. _____
_____

3. _____
_____

■ ■
■ Starting lineup

Although an implanted port is surgically placed by a doctor, you may need to assist or provide preoperative or postoperative patient care. Put these steps in the proper sequence to show that you know what this procedure entails.

A subcutaneous pocket is made over a bony prominence on the chest wall, and the catheter is tunneled to the pocket.	
A small incision is made, and the catheter is introduced into the superior vena cava through the subclavian, jugular, or cephalic vein.	
The reservoir is sutured to the underlying fascia, and the incision is closed.	
The catheter is connected to the port reservoir, which is placed in the pocket and flushed with heparinized saline solution.	
A dressing is applied to the wound site.	
Fluoroscopy is used to verify placement of the catheter tip.	

Boxing match

Part of your care for a patient undergoing port implantation involves patient teaching. Fill in the answers to the clues below by using all of the syllables in the box. The number of syllables for each answer is shown in parentheses. Use each syllable only once.

A	CON	FIL	FORMED	GRAM	HEP	I
IN	IN	LAC	~~MOVE~~	~~MENT~~	O	PRO
PHY	~~RE~~	RIN	SENT	~~STRIC~~	TIC	TION
TION	~~TIONS~~	TRA	VEN	ZA		

1. Knowing these beforehand will gain the patient's cooperation with lying still during the procedure

   (5) M O V E M E N T
        R E S T R I C T I O N S

2. An X-ray picture of the patient's blood flow that's helpful in determining the best vessel to use

   (3) _ _ _ _ _ _ _

3. A legal document required by most facilities before a patient undergoes an invasive procedure

   (4) _ _ _ _ _ _ _
        _ _ _ _ _ _

4. The name given to antibiotics taken before a surgical or dental procedure to prevent contamination and colonization of the implanted port

   (4) _ _ _ _ _ _ _ _ _ _ _

5. Leaking or seepage of irritating medication, which can damage the tissue surrounding a port if not quickly treated; signs and symptoms include pain and swelling at the site

   (4) _ _ _ _ _ _ _ _ _ _ _

6. Flushing procedure required to maintain patency and prevent occlusion of the port and infusion equipment; the patient or a family member may be taught how to do this

   (6) _ _ _ _ _ _ _ _ _ _ _ _

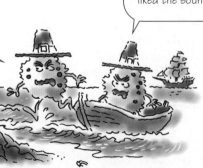

After we've cleared the harbor and set foot on that large rock, we'll declare this new land "Implanted Port."

Whatever happened to "Massachusetts?" I liked the sound of that.

■ Mind sprints

For 7 to 10 days following port implantation, you'll need to monitor the patient for signs of five potential problems. See if you can list all five of these signs in 1 minute or less.

- _____
- _____
- _____
- _____
- _____

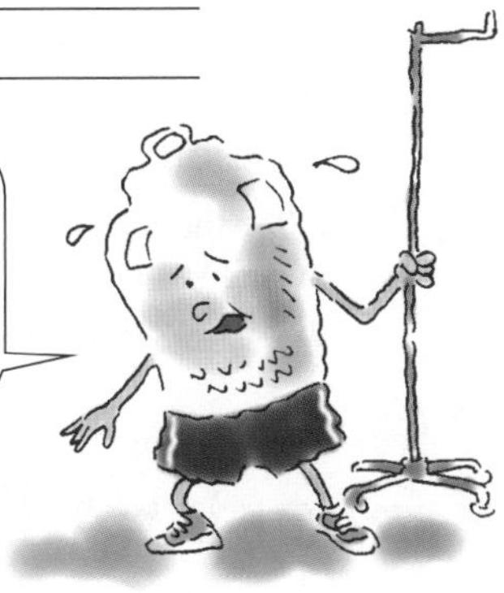

I'm glad all I have to do is hang out and relax during the actual infusion—all this preparation is quite a workout!

■ Starting lineup

Show that you know how to prepare infusion equipment when using an implanted port by putting the following steps in proper sequence.

Prime the noncoring needle and extension set with saline solution from the syringe. (Prime the tubing and purge it of air using strict aseptic technique.)	
Attach the tubing to the solution container.	
If setting up an intermittent system, fill two syringes— one with 10 ml of normal saline solution and the other with 5 ml of heparin solution (100 units/ml).	
After priming the tubing, recheck all connections for tightness. Make sure that all open ends are covered with sealed caps.	
Prime the tubing with fluid.	

Pep talk

❝ For true success ask yourself these four questions: Why? Why not? Why not me? Why not now? ❞

—Jimmy Dean

■■
■ Hit or miss

Mark the statements about administering a bolus injection by implanted port with a "T" for "True" and an "F" for "False."

_____ 1. You should begin by attaching a 10-ml syringe filled with saline solution to the end of an extension set, and remove all the air; then attach the extension set to a noncoring needle.

_____ 2. You should always check for a blood return; then flush the port with a saline solution followed by heparin solution, following facility policy.

_____ 3. You should always clamp the extension set when changing syringes after flushing.

_____ 4. It's important to check for fever, nausea, vomiting, leukocytosis, malaise, and elevated glucose level during a bolus injection, as these are signs and symptoms of infiltration.

_____ 5. After the injection, you should clamp the extension set and remove the medication syringe; then flush with 5 ml of saline solution, followed by heparin solution, according to facility policy.

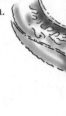

I love these saline flushes… wheeee!

■■
■ Starting lineup

Put these steps in sequence to show you know how to safely and securely access a top-entry implanted port.

Flush the device with normal saline solution. If you detect swelling or the patient complains of pain, remove the needle and notify the practitioner.	
Anchor the port between your thumb and the first two fingers of your nondominant hand. Then, using your dominant hand, aim the needle at the center of the device, between your thumb and first finger.	
If you can't obtain blood, remove the needle and repeat the procedure. If you still can't obtain a blood return, notify the practitioner immediately.	
With the patient sitting upright and with his back supported, palpate the area over the port to locate the septum.	
Check the needle placement by aspirating for a blood return.	
Insert the needle perpendicular to the port septum. Push the needle through the skin and septum until you reach the bottom of the reservoir (you'll feel the back of the port).	

■■
■ Mind sprints

The practitioner may order a thrombolytic agent when a patient's implanted port is compromised by a suspected clot. As quick as you can, list at least five conditions in which treatment with a thrombolytic is contraindicated.

- _____
- _____
- _____
- _____
- _____

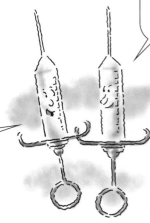

> I guess we'll be putting in a little overtime tonight.

■■
■ Starting lineup

> Looks like there might be a clot holding up the works.

Put the following steps in sequence to indicate the proper procedure for clearing an implanted port and catheter using a prescribed thrombolytic agent when the patient has a suspected clot.

Check for a blood return.

Attach the syringe containing the prescribed thrombolytic agent and unclamp the extension tubing.

Clamp the extension set, and leave the solution in place for 15 minutes (up to 30 minutes in some facilities).

Palpate the area over the port, and then access the port.

Instill the thrombolytic using a gentle pull-push motion on the syringe plunger to mix the solution in the access equipment, port, and catheter.

Flush the port with 5 ml of saline solution, and clamp the extension tubing.

Attach an empty 10-ml syringe, unclamp the extension set, and aspirate the thrombolytic and clot with the 10-ml syringe; then discard the syringe. If the clot can't be aspirated, wait 15 minutes before trying again.

After the blockage is cleared, flush the catheter with at least 10 ml of saline solution, and then flush with heparin solution.

■ Match point

Knowing how to deal with common implanted port problems is part of port maintenance. Match the implanted port problem on the left with the nursing intervention on the right.

Implanted port problem

1. Kinked catheter, catheter migration, or port rotation _____
2. Kinked tubing or closed clamp _____
3. Incorrect needle placement or needle that won't advance through septum _____
4. Deeply implanted port _____
5. Clot formation _____

Nursing intervention

A. Regain access to the device; teach the home care patient to push down firmly on the noncoring needle device in the septum and aspirate for blood return.

B. Assess patency by trying to flush the port while the patient changes position; notify the practitioner and obtain an order for a thrombolytic; teach the patient to recognize signs and symptoms, notify the practitioner, and avoid forcibly flushing the port.

C. Notify the practitioner immediately; tell the patient to notify the practitioner immediately if he has trouble using the implanted port.

D. Check the equipment.

E. Note the portal chamber scar; use deep palpation; ask another nurse for help; use a 1″ to 2″ noncoring needle to gain access to the port.

■ Starting lineup

Show that you understand how to discontinue implanted port therapy by putting the following steps in their proper sequence.

Remove the noncoring needle, and dispose of it properly.	
After shutting off the infusion, clamp the extension set and remove the I.V. tubing.	
Gather the necessary equipment: a 10-ml syringe filled with 5 ml of normal saline solution, a 10-ml syringe filled with 5 ml of sterile heparin flush solution (100 units/ml), sterile gloves, sterile 2″ × 2″ gauze pad, and tape.	
Attach the syringe filled with saline solution using aseptic technique.	
Unclamp the extension set, flush the device with saline solution, and remove the saline solution syringe.	
Attach the heparin syringe, flush the port with the heparin solution, and clamp the extension set.	
Document the procedure and your findings.	

Jumble gym

Preventing complications of implanted port therapy is an important part of your routine nursing management. Use the clues to help you unscramble common port-related complications. Then use the circled letters to answer the question posed.

Question: Prevention of what complication includes flushing the port right after obtaining a blood sample and administering packed red blood cells as a piggyback solution with saline solution?

1. Characterized by fever, redness, swelling, oozing or purulent drainage, and warmth at the port site

K N S I   N O N F T I C I E   ◯ _ _ _   _ _ _ _ _ ◯ _ ◯ _

2. May be helped by warm soaks applied for 20 minutes four times per day

K N I S   D A R K B W E O N   _ _ _ _   ◯ _ _ _ _ _ ◯ _ _

3. Causes a burning sensation or swelling in subcutaneous tissue, often resulting from needle displacement or catheter rupture

V E T O X I N S A R A T A   _ _ _ ◯ _ _ _ ◯ _ _ _ _ _

4. Caused by adherence of platelets to the catheter and may require instillation of a thrombolytic

I B N F I R   E T H A H S   T O M F R A N I O
_ _ _ ◯ _   _ _ _ _ _ ◯   _ _ _ ◯ _ _ _ _

Answer: _ _ _ _ _ _ _ _ _ _

Starting lineup

Show that you know the safe way to remove a noncoring needle following an infusion by putting the following steps in the proper sequence.

Place the gloved index and middle fingers from the nondominant hand on either side of the port septum.
Apply a dressing as indicated.
Stabilize the port by pressing down with the index and middle fingers, maintaining pressure until the needle is removed.
If no more infusions are scheduled, remind the patient that he'll need a heparin flush in 4 weeks.
Put on gloves.
Using your gloved, dominant hand, grasp the noncoring needle and pull it straight out of the port.

■■
■ Batter's box

Never forget the importance of documenting your assessment findings and interventions throughout a patient's entire port therapy. Fill in the blanks with answers from the options listed below. Use each option only once.

Always record your assessment findings and interventions according to your

_____ . Be sure to include such information as the:

1

- type, amount, rate, and _____ of the infusion

2

- appearance of the _____

3

- development of _____ , as well as the steps taken to resolve them

4

- type of needle used, including its _____ and length

5

- type of _____ changes for continuous infusions

6

- _____ samples obtained, including type and amount

7

- _____ topics covered

8

- patient's response to all _____ .

9

After removing the noncoring needle, remember to document the:

- _____ of the infusion needle and status of the site

10

- use of _____ flush

11

- patient's _____ of the procedure

12

- your teaching efforts

- any problems encountered and resolved.

Options
A. blood
B. dressing
C. duration
D. facility's policy
E. gauge
F. heparin
G. patient-teaching
H. problems
I. procedures
J. removal
K. site
L. tolerance

Remember, thorough documentation of all I.V. procedures, complications, and patient teaching efforts can protect you and your practice.

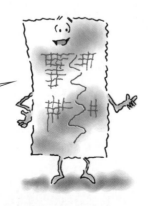

4

I.V. medications

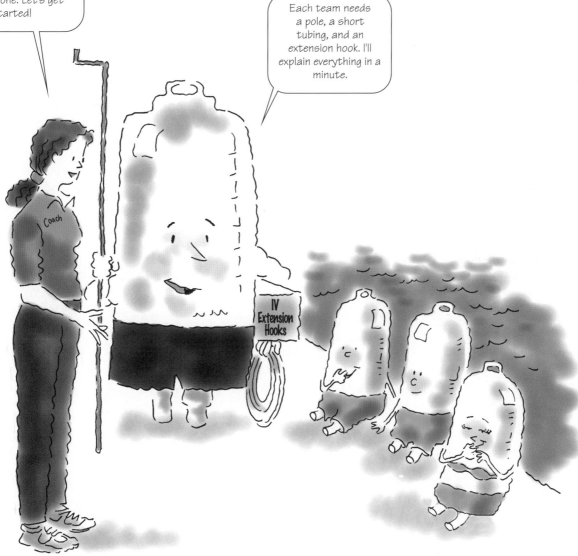

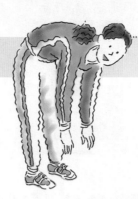

I.V. medications review

Benefits

- Achieve rapid therapeutic drug levels
- Are absorbed more effectively than drugs given by other routes
- Permit accurate titration
- Produce less discomfort

Risks

- May cause solution and drug incompatibilities
- May lead to poor vascular access
- Can produce immediate adverse reactions

I.V. administration methods

I.V. bolus injection

- Drug injected through an existing I.V. line
- Drug injected slowly (unless specified) to prevent adverse reactions and vein trauma

Intermittent infusion

- Drug administered over a specified interval
- Drug delivered through a piggyback line, saline lock, or volume-control set

Continuous infusion

- Drug delivery regulated over an extended time
- Drug delivered through a primary or secondary line

PCA therapy

- Referred to as *patient-controlled analgesia* (PCA)
- Overdose prevented by lock-out interval
- Patient uses fewer opioids for pain relief

Monitoring

- Patient monitored for respiratory depression
- Patient monitored for decreased blood pressure

Assessment

- Pain relief (frequently)
- Infiltration into surrounding tissues

Potential complications

- Hypersensitivity
- Infiltration
- Extravasation
- Phlebitis
- Infection

■ ■
■ Mind sprints

Hospitalized patients receive about 50% of their medications by the I.V. route.
In 30 seconds or less, list the three ways by which I.V. medications are delivered.

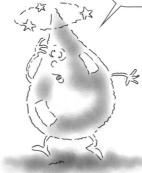

> About half of all medications given to hospitalized patients are given I.V. It makes my head spin just to think about it!

■ _____

■ _____

■ _____

■ ■
■ Batter's box

Fill in the blanks with the correct information regarding I.V. medications.

An I.V. medication may be ordered when:

■ a patient needs a rapid _____ effect
  1

■ the medication can't be absorbed by the _____ , either because it
  2

  has a high _____ or is affected by high _____ acidity
  3   4

■ the patient may receive nothing by _____ and an irritating drug
  5

  would cause _____ or tissue damage if given I.M. or
  6

  _____ (also called *subQ*)
  7

■ a controlled _____ is needed.
  8

Options
A. administration rate
B. gastric
C. GI tract
D. molecular weight
E. mouth
F. pain
G. subcutaneously
H. therapeutic

Pep talk

❝ Logic will get you from A to B. Imagination will take you everywhere.
—Albert Einstein ❞

Hit or miss

Mark each statement about the benefits of I.V. drug administration with a "T" for "True" or an "F" for "False."

_____ 1. I.V. drugs may be given to an uncooperative patient, but they shouldn't be given to a patient who's unconscious.

_____ 2. I.V. medications go directly into the patient's circulation, rapidly achieving therapeutic effects.

_____ 3. In the event of an adverse reaction, I.V. drug delivery can be stopped immediately.

_____ 4. Medications given I.V. are absorbed at the same rate as those given subQ or I.M.

_____ 5. The I.V. route may be the best alternative when an oral drug is poorly absorbed due to unstable gastric juices and digestive enzymes.

_____ 6. The I.V. route allows for accurate titration of drug doses because gastric absorption isn't a problem.

_____ 7. With I.V. medications, accurate titration is achieved by adjusting the concentration and temperature of the infusate.

_____ 8. Venous irritation may be reduced by diluting an I.V. medication in a smaller volume of solute.

Train your brain

Sound out each group of pictures and symbols to reveal important information about I.V. drug administration.

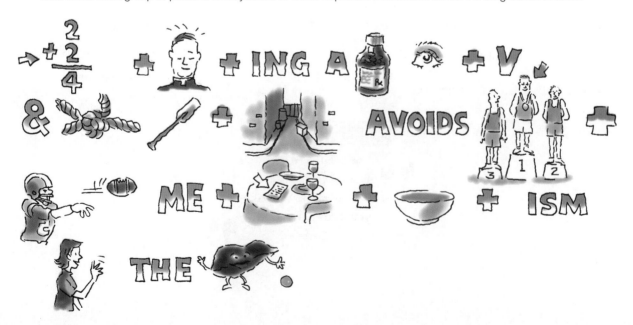

Power stretch

Stretch your knowledge of risks to I.V. drug therapy by first unscrambling the words on the left to reveal three types of drug and solution incompatibilities. Then draw a line from the box to its multiple description, characteristics, and examples on the right.

YASHLIPC

— — — — — — — —

CLICAMHE

— — — — — — — —

UCTARTIPEHE

— — — — — — — — — —

A. Alters the integrity and potency of active ingredients when two drugs are mixed

B. Can be prevented by administering drugs at different times

C. Occurs when heparin is mixed with an aminoglycoside infusion

D. Occurs when calcium is mixed with another drug

E. May be affected by drug concentration, pH, volume, or exposure to light

F. Also called a *pharmaceutical incompatibility*

G. Occurs when two or more drugs are administered concurrently

H. Occurs when chloramphenicol and penicillin are mixed

I. Commonly occurs with multiple additives

Strikeout

These statements pertain to drug and solution incompatibilities. Cross out all of the incorrect statements.

1. To successfully mix medication in a solution for infusion, the drug and diluent must be compatible.

2. Very few I.V. drugs are compatible with commonly used I.V. solutions.

3. The more complex the solution, the less risk exists for incompatibility.

4. An I.V. solution containing divalent cations (such as calcium) has a lower incidence of incompatibility.

5. Incompatibility problems are common in mixtures containing other electrolytes, mannitol, bicarbonate, or nutritional solutions.

I've looked into those online dating services, but nothing beats a good old-fashioned drug compatibility chart.

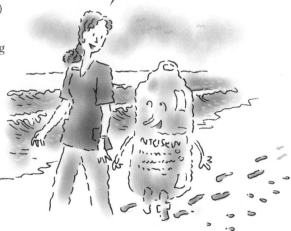

Match point

Several factors can affect the chemical compatibility of I.V. drugs or solutions that are mixed together. Match the factor (on the left) with the reason why a chemical reaction might occur (on the right).

Factor

1. Light _____
2. Contact time _____
3. Temperature _____
4. Order of mixing _____
5. Drug concentration _____
6. pH _____

Reason

A. Chemical changes occur after each drug is added to a solution; a drug that's compatible with the I.V. solution alone might be incompatible with the mixture of the I.V. solution and another drug.

B. Prolonged exposure can affect the stability of certain drugs.

C. Drugs and solutions that aren't within the same range of acidity or alkalinity may cause an undesirable chemical reaction when mixed.

D. Heat promotes chemical reactions, increasing the risk of incompatibilities.

E. The longer two or more drugs are together, the more likely an incompatibility will occur.

F. Buildup of a large amount of one drug in a solution can cause an incompatibility with other drugs in the solution; drugs should be evenly dispersed before infusion.

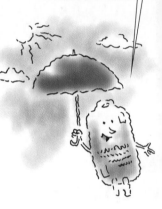

As long as I'm clamped, I don't mind a little rain. But too much bright light can be a big problem.

Boxing match

Fill in the answers to the clues to identify four reasons why normally accessible veins could collapse or become small and scarred and, therefore, unsuitable for I.V. drug administration. The number of syllables for each answer appears in parentheses. Use each syllable only once.

A	CON	HY	IR	LE	MI	NI	PEA
PO	PUNC	RE	RI	SO	STRIC	TA	TED
TING	TION	TURES	VA	VE	VO		

1. Narrowing of a blood vessel caused by contraction of the vessel's muscles

(5) __ __ __ __ __ __ __ __ __ __ __ __ __ __

2. Decreased blood volume

(6) __ __ __ __ __ __ __ __ __ __ __

3. Often required when a patient needs frequent or prolonged I.V. therapy

(7) __ __ __ __ __ __ __ __ __

__ __ __ __ __ __ __ __ __ __ __ __ __

4. Infusion of these types of drugs

(4) __ __ __ __ __ __ __ __ __

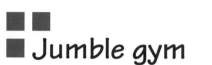

Jumble gym

Use the clues to help you guess these terms related to adverse drug reactions. Then use the circled letters to answer the question posed.

Question: Besides the drug's active ingredient, which chemical substances can cause severe reactions, especially in neonates and patients with asthma?

1. Undesirable reaction that can develop immediately or anytime after administration of an I.V. drug; can range from mild to severe or even lethal

_ _ ◯ _ _ _ ◯ _ _ _ _ _ ◯ _ _ _

2. Adverse reaction stemming from an inherent inability to tolerate certain chemicals; can cause effects opposite those expected

_ _ _ _ ◯ _ _ _ _ _ ◯ _ _   ◯◯ _ _ _ _ _ _

3. Severe, life-threatening allergic reaction to a drug; may develop very quickly after administration of a drug

◯ _ _ _ _ _ _ _ ◯◯

4. Adverse reaction to a chemically similar drug or group of drugs

_ ◯ _ _ _ - _ ◯ _ _ _ _ _ ◯ _ _ _

Answer: _ _ _ _ _ _ _ _ _ _ _ _ _

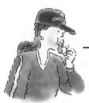

Coaching session
Recognizing anaphylaxis

Although hypersensitivity to I.V. drugs is relatively uncommon, these type of reactions can develop immediately or anytime after administration. Anaphylaxis, the most severe form of hypersensitivity, is life-threatening and requires prompt treatment.

Common signs and symptoms of a drug-related anaphylaxis reaction include:
- respiratory distress (bronchospasm, stridor, decreased air movement)
- skin changes (cyanosis, urticaria, angioedema, cold, clammy skin)
- cardiovascular problems (tachycardia, hypotension, arrhythmias, chest pain)
- central nervous system changes (dizziness, anxiety, decreased sensorium, loss of consciousness).

■ Mind sprints

In many cases, you must calculate an ordered dosage and verify that the dosage is within the recommended range. In 1 minute or less, list the two measures on which most dosages are based.

■ _____

■ _____

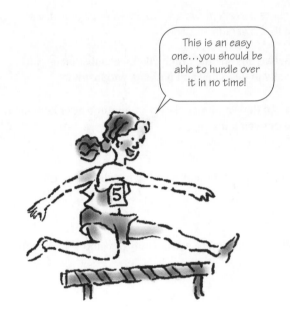

This is an easy one...you should be able to hurdle over it in no time!

■ Hit or miss

Mark each statement about calculating I.V. drug dosages and administration rates with a "T" for "True" and an "F" for "False."

_____ 1. To convert a patient's weight from pounds to kilograms, you should simply multiply the number by 2.2.

_____ 2. Dosages of chemotherapeutic drugs are commonly based on the patient's body surface area (BSA).

_____ 3. Typically, an order for I.V. medication states the number of milliliters to infuse over a specified period.

_____ 4. Additional I.V. orders should have no effect on your original calculations for a drug.

You make the call

Identify the calculation tools illustrated here, and briefly describe how they're used.

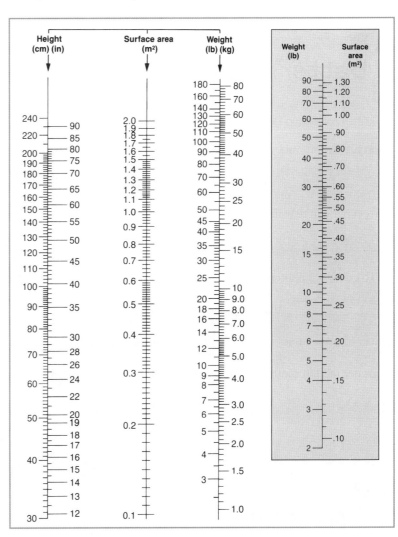

Calculation tool: _____
_____

Calculation tool: _____
_____

How they're used: _____
_____
_____
_____

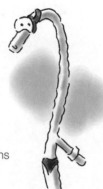

Make sure your calculations are correct based on the type of I.V. equipment you're using.

Batter's box

Use the options to fill in the missing information about equipment considerations when calculating I.V. drug administration.

Your calculations may depend on the delivery equipment. If you're using an

_____ , simply set the machine for the desired rate of _____ .
$\quad$ 1 $\qquad\qquad\qquad\qquad\qquad\qquad$ 2

However, if you're using an administration set, you have to convert milliliters per hour to

_____ .
$\quad$ 3

$\quad$ To convert milliliters per hour to drops per minute, you must know the number of

_____ that the particular I.V. tubing delivers. _____ tubings
$\quad$ 4 $\qquad\qquad\qquad\qquad\qquad$ 5

deliver 60 gtt/ml, but _____ tubings vary in their delivery rates. To find
$\qquad\qquad\qquad\qquad$ 6

drops per milliliter information, check the product wrapper or box; then use this formula:

$$\underset{7}{\underline{\hspace{3cm}}} \text{ in drops/minute} = \frac{\text{total milliliters}}{\text{total minutes}} \times \underset{8}{\underline{\hspace{3cm}}} \text{ in drops/ml}$$

Options

A. drip rate

B. drop factor

C. drops per milliliter

D. drops per minute

E. infusion pump

F. macrodrip

G. microdrip

H. milliliters per hour

Strikeout

These statements pertain to basic safety measures that are needed when preparing a medication for I.V. administration. Cross out the incorrect statements.

1. You should always maintain clean technique when administering I.V. medications.

2. You should always wash your hands before mixing a drug, and avoid contaminating any part of the vial, ampule, syringe, needleless adapter, or container that must remain sterile.

3. To avoid contaminating the adapter with your finger when inserting and withdrawing a needleless adapter into a vial, you should keep your hands steady and brace one hand against the other.

4. When drawing up a drug before adding it to the primary solution, you should always use two syringes to hold the entire dose.

Team colors

Draw a red line on the nomogram to calculate the BSA of a patient with the following statistical information. Then write the patient's BSA in the space provided.

Question: The patient's height is 5′ 9″ (175 cm) and his weight is 178 lb (80.7 kg). The patient's BSA is _____ .

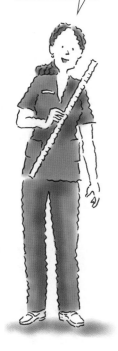

Always measure carefully and strive for accuracy!

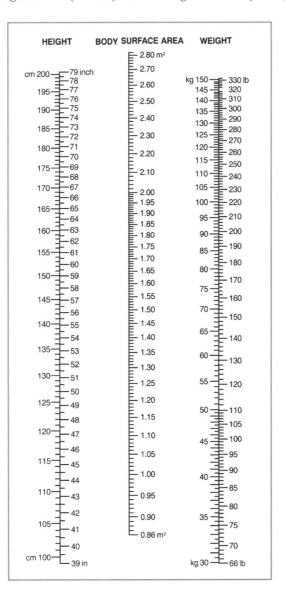

■ Match point

Reconstituting a drug is sometimes necessary before the drug can be administered. Show you know which constituents to use by matching each term on the left with its description on the right.

Term

1. Diluent _____
2. Reconstitution _____
3. Solution _____
4. Admixture _____
5. Microcontainer _____

Description

A. Homogeneous mixture of two or more substances

B. Small bag or bottle that holds liquid used for reconstituting drugs

C. Liquid used to reconstitute drug that's in powdered form; examples include normal saline solution, sterile water for injection, and dextrose 5% in water

D. Solution produced after mixing a powdered drug with a diluent

E. Restoration of a powdered drug to its liquid state

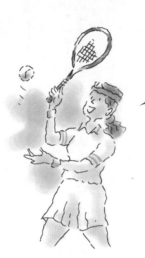

After this workout, I was planning to reconstitute some powdered margarita mix. Care to join me?

■ Hit or miss

Mark each statement about reconstituting drugs with a "T" for "True" or an "F" for "False."

_____ 1. It's unnecessary to check the expiration date on diluents because such solutions are made with sterile water.

_____ 2. Some drugs require filtration during the reconstitution process.

_____ 3. Before reconstitution, you should always inspect the drug, diluent, and solution for particles and cloudiness.

_____ 4. If no particles or cloudiness are noted before reconstitution, there's no need to check the admixture afterward because all of the constituents were obviously pure.

_____ 5. It's important to know that most drugs are moderately alkaline.

_____ 6. Some solutions used as diluents change color after several hours in a microcontainer, so it's best to check with the pharmacist if you're unsure whether to use them.

■ Starting lineup

Show that you know how to safely reconstitute powdered drugs by putting the following steps in the correct sequence.

Check for visible signs of incompatibility once the drug is fully reconstituted.	
Connect the syringe to the needleless adapter on the vial.	
Inject the diluent into the drug vial.	
Draw up the amount and type of diluent specified by the manufacturer.	
Mix the solution by gently rotating the vial.	
Clean the rubber stopper of the drug vial with an alcohol swab, using aseptic technique.	
Watch to ensure that the powder is thoroughly dissolved. If it isn't fully dissolved, let the vial stand for 10 to 30 minutes; if necessary, agitate it several times gently to dissolve the drug.	

■ Mind sprints

Liquid drugs don't need reconstitution, but they often need to be diluted before I.V. administration. In 1 minute or less, list four ways you would expect liquid medications to be packaged for use on the nursing unit.

■ _____

■ _____

■ _____

■ _____

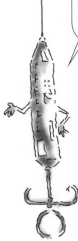

The point is, there are only a few ways to conveniently package liquid medication for ready use.

■ Starting lineup

You can add a drug to an I.V. bottle or bag or, when necessary, to an I.V. solution that's already infusing. Show that you know the correct way to add a drug by putting these steps in their proper sequence.

Adding to an I.V. bottle

Invert the bottle at least twice to ensure thorough mixing.	
Clean the rubber stopper or latex diaphragm with alcohol.	
Remove the latex diaphragm, and insert the administration spike.	
Attach the needleless adapter and the medication-filled syringe into the center of the stopper or diaphragm, and inject the drug.	

Adding to a plastic I.V. bag

Grasp the top and bottom of the bag, and quickly invert it twice.	
Attach the needleless adapter and the medication-filled syringe into the clean latex medication port.	
Inject the drug.	

Adding to an infusing I.V. solution bag

Clean the rubber injection port with an alcohol swab.	
Make sure the primary solution container has enough solution to provide adequate dilution.	
Inject the drug, keeping the container upright.	
Clamp the I.V. tubing, and take down the container.	

Match point

When choosing equipment for I.V. drug administration, you must consider the choice of drug, equipment features and limitations, and the patient's specific needs. Match the equipment on the left with its special consideration on the right.

Equipment

1. I.V. delivery pump _____
2. Microdrip tubing _____
3. Nonvented tubing _____
4. Tubing with backcheck valve _____
5. Tubing with injection port close to the venipuncture device _____
6. Tubing without polyvinyl chloride _____
7. Vented I.V. tubing _____
8. Volume-control infusion set _____

Special consideration

A. Used with a collapsible plastic I.V. solution bag

B. Needed when the infusion rate is less than 63 ml/hour

C. Used when you need a precise or very low infusion rate

D. Needed for giving simultaneous infusions

E. Used with a glass I.V. solution container

F. Recommended when giving such drugs as nitroglycerin or paclitaxel

G. Often required when administering I.V. drugs to infants or small children

H. Needed for giving intermittent infusions

You make the call

Identify the type of equipment illustrated here. Then describe the specific areas highlighted.

> Take it from me: choosing the right equipment can make all the difference in your I.V. game plan.

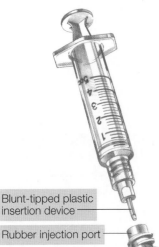

Blunt-tipped plastic insertion device

Rubber injection port

Type of equipment: _____

Describe the highlighted areas: _____

_____

_____

_____

_____

Memory jogger

Before administering an I.V. drug to a patient, always remember to check the five **rights**:

- _____
- _____
- _____
- _____
- _____

■ Hit or miss

Mark each statement about the direct injection method of medication infusion with a "T" for "True" or an "F" for "False."

_____ 1. An I.V. bolus injection, also known as an *I.V. push*, can be used to give a bolus (single dose) or intermittent multiple doses.

_____ 2. To avoid speed shock, drugs given by I.V. bolus are typically administered over 1 minute or more.

_____ 3. Even emergency drugs, such as those used to treat cardiac or respiratory arrest, are given over 1 minute or longer when administered by I.V. bolus.

_____ 4. Patients with systemic edema, pulmonary congestion, decreased cardiac output, or reduced urine output, renal flow, or glomerular filtration rate sometimes require a faster injection time or more concentrated drugs to decrease drug tolerance.

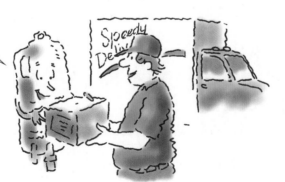

They sure weren't kidding about bolus deliveries guaranteed in 1 minute or less. I think I'm still in speed shock!

Pep talk

" Any human anywhere will blossom in a hundred unexpected talents and capacities simply by being given the opportunity to do so.

—Doris Lessing "

■■
■ Finish line

A volume-control device may be used as part of an intermittent set to deliver I.V. medications. Identify the equipment shown in this illustration.

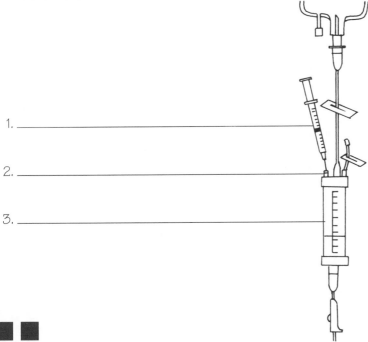

1. _____

2. _____

3. _____

■■
■ Power stretch

Stretch your knowledge of I.V. medications by first unscrambling the words on the left to reveal three ways in which drugs are given by intermittent infusion. Then draw a line from the box to the specific advantages of using each method on the right. (Note that each entry will have more than one advantage.)

BIGPAYKGC
MODHET

_ _ _ _ _ _ _ _ _

_ _ _ _ _ _ _

LEANSI CLOK

_ _ _ _ _ _   _ _ _ _

MUVELO-RNOOLTC
STE

_ _ _ _ _ _ _ - _ _ _ _ _ _ _ _

_ _ _

A. Provides venous access for patients with fluid restrictions

B. Provides high drug blood levels for short periods without causing drug toxicity

C. Requires only one large-volume container

D. Allows the chamber to be reused

E. Preserves veins by reducing venipunctures

F. Avoids multiple needle injections required by I.M. route

G. Permits repeated administration of drugs through a single I.V. site

H. Prevents fluid overload from a runaway infusion

I. Provides better patient mobility between doses

J. Lowers cost if used with a limited number of drugs

■■
■ Batter's box

Fill in the blanks with answers from the options below to complete the information about piggyback infusions.

After setting up the equipment, lower the primary infusion with the supplied

_____ below the level of the _____ container. Then open the
     1   2

_____ of the secondary set, and allow the medication to infuse as prescribed.
     3

Because the secondary container hangs higher than the primary container, fluid flowing

from it creates pressure on the _____ and completely shuts off fluid flow
                                          4

from the primary container. The primary infusion will restart automatically once the

secondary infusion is completed.

If the _____ doesn't have a backcheck valve, you must clamp the primary
               5

line (lowering the primary line isn't necessary). After the piggyback infusion is completed,

open the clamp to prevent the venous access device from _____ .
                                                6

Options

A. backcheck valve

B. clogging

C. extension hook

D. flow clamp

E. primary tubing

F. secondary medication

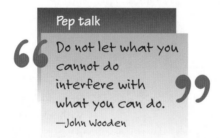

Pep talk

" Do not let what you cannot do interfere with what you can do. "
—John Wooden

Finish line

This illustration shows the components needed for an intermittent piggyback infusion. Identify each piece of equipment highlighted.

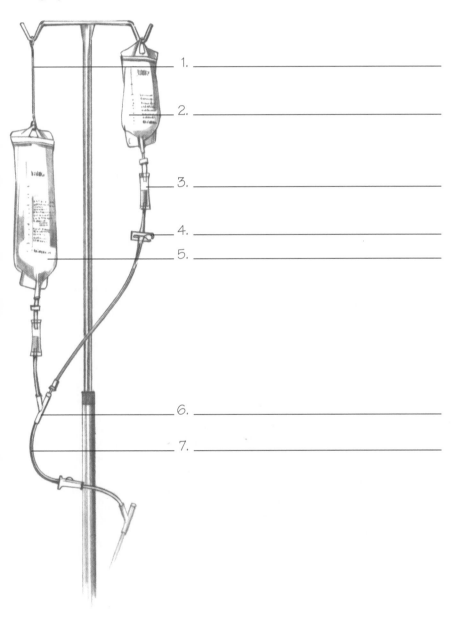

1. _____

2. _____

3. _____

4. _____

5. _____

6. _____

7. _____

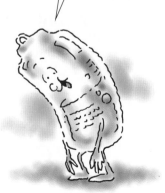

Always check my back—my backcheck valve, that is—if you're using a piggyback system. If it's missing, you'll need to clamp my primary line before running a secondary line.

■■ Starting lineup

Put these steps in the correct order to show how you would safely administer a medication using a saline lock with an intermittent infusion set.

Clean the cap on the saline lock with an alcohol swab.	
Attach the minibag to the administration set, and prime the tubing with the drug solution.	
Stabilize the saline lock with the thumb and index finger of your nondominant hand.	
Regulate the drip rate, and infuse the medication as ordered.	
Insert the needleless device of a syringe containing flush solution into the center of the injection cap; then pull back the plunger slightly to watch for a blood return, and slowly inject the flush solution.	
Secure a needleless device to the I.V. tubing, and prime the device with the drug solution.	
Insert the needleless device attached to the administration set into the saline lock.	

■■ You make the call

Using the space provided, briefly describe the procedure shown here and explain why it's important.

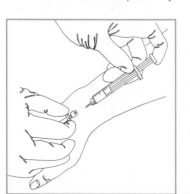

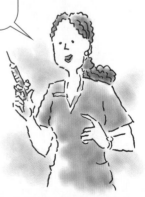

Don't forget, when administering drugs with a saline lock, you'll need to use two 3-ml syringes filled with saline flush solution—one before injecting the medication, the other after discontinuing the infusion.

_____

_____

_____

_____

_____

■ Hit or miss

Mark each statement about administering drugs through a volume-control device with a "T" for "True" or an "F" for "False."

_____ 1. You can use a volume-control set as either a primary or secondary line.

_____ 2. After adding medication to the volume-control chamber, you should immediately write the drug, dose, time, and date directly on the chamber in ink.

_____ 3. You should fill the chamber with the prescribed amount of solution to dilute the medication; then vigorously shake the device to thoroughly mix the medication and solution.

_____ 4. You should always check for an immediately visible incompatibility after adding medications to a volume-control set, especially if you're using multiple lines.

_____ 5. If you're using a volume-control set as a secondary line, you should remember to stop the primary infusion or set it at a low drip rate so the line will be open when the secondary infusion is completed.

_____ 6. After the infusion and if the patient can tolerate extra fluid, you should open the upper clamp and let 10 ml of I.V. solution to flow into the chamber and through the tubing to flush it and complete delivery of the medication.

■ Starting lineup

Show that you know how to prime a volume-control set by putting these steps in the correct sequence.

Release the drip chamber.
Fill the chamber with 20 ml of fluid.
Close the regulating clamp directly below the drip chamber.
Squeeze and hold the drip chamber.
Open the flow-regulating clamp.

■ Boxing match

Fill in the answers to the clues about continuous I.V. medication infusions by using all of the syllables in the boxes. The number of syllables for each answer is shown in parentheses. Use each syllable only once.

DOSE	E	ELS	FLU	ID	IN	ING	LEC	LEV
LIN	LOAD	LOAD	LYTE	O	SU	TRO	VER	

1. May be needed before starting a continuous infusion to achieve peak serum levels quickly

   (3) __ __ __ __ __ __ __ __ __ __

2. May enhance the effectiveness of some drugs, such as heparin and this

   (3) __ __ __ __ __ __ __

3. May result from receiving too much I.V. solution; can be prevented by maintaining accurate intake and output records and weighing the patient daily

   (5) __ __ __ __ __ __ __ __ __ __ __ __ __

4. May cause significant physiologic changes if not within normal limits; require careful monitoring of laboratory results

   (6) __ __ __ __ __ __ __ __ __ __ __ __

   __ __ __ __ __ __

■ Batter's box

Complete this information about PCA by filling in answers using the options below.

PCA therapy allows your patient to control I.V. therapy of an _____
                                                                    1

(usually _____) and maintain therapeutic _____ of the drug.
              2   3

The computerized PCA pump delivers medication through an I.V. administration set that's

attached directly to the patient's I.V. line; the patient receives a dose of medication by

pushing a button on a _____ . A _____ prevents the patient
                              4   5

from accidentally overdosing by imposing a _____ between doses—usually
                                                    6

6 to 10 minutes.

   PCA therapy is commonly used by patients after _____ and by patients
                                                            7

with chronic diseases, particularly those with terminal _____ or
                                                                8

_____ .
       9

Options

A. analgesic

B. cancer

C. hand-held controller

D. lock-out time

E. morphine

F. serum levels

G. sickle cell disease

H. surgery

I. timing unit

Match point

Match the PCA-related problem on the left with its corresponding nursing intervention on the right.

PCA-related problem

1. Constipation _____

2. Enhanced central nervous system (CNS) depression _____

3. Nausea _____

4. Respiratory depression _____

5. Overdose _____

6. Poor ventilation and pooling of secretions _____

7. Orthostatic hypotension _____

Nursing intervention

A. Instruct the patient to breathe deeply; if he's confused, stop the infusion and prepare to administer oxygen.

B. Instruct the patient to eat a high-fiber diet, drink plenty of fluids, and take a stool softener.

C. Assess for slow or irregular breathing, pinpoint pupils, and loss of consciousness.

D. Encourage the patient to practice coughing and deep breathing.

E. Instruct the patient to rise slowly from a supine or sitting position

F. Caution the patient against drinking alcohol.

G. Administer an antiemetic, such as chlorpromazine.

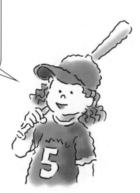

When it comes to giving I.V. drugs, remember that infants, elderly patients, and kids like me have special fluid requirements— a little bit can go a long way!

Hit or miss

Mark each statement about administering I.V. medications to pediatric and elderly patients with a "T" for "True" or an "F" for "False."

_____ 1. Pediatric dosages are based largely on the age of the child.

_____ 2. Elderly patients have fragile veins and are prone to many I.V.-related problems.

_____ 3. The most common method of giving I.V. drugs to pediatric patients is by I.V. bolus.

_____ 4. When using a volume-control pump on a pediatric patient, you should choose one with an anti-free-flow device to prevent inadvertent bolus infusions in case the pump is accidentally opened.

_____ 5. Elderly patients are especially prone to infiltration, phlebitis, and fluid overload.

_____ 6. When administering an I.V. analgesic to an elderly patient, you should watch closely for increased respirations and CNS excitation.

■ Cross-training

Recognizing and promptly treating complications is critical when administering I.V. medications. Complete this crossword puzzle to test your knowledge of what to look for and what to do.

Across

3. This complication causes itching, rash, runny nose, tearing, and breathing difficulty.

4. This complication causes redness or tenderness at the tip of the device, a puffy area over the vein, and an elevated temperature.

7. Semi-Fowler's position, oxygen, and diuretics may correct this complication. (Two words)

8. Remove the I.V. device, elevate the limb, check the pulse and capillary refill, and reinsert the infusion device if this complication isn't too serious.

10. When you encounter this complication, apply warm soaks over the vein and surrounding tissue, then slow the flow rate (which could be sluggish if the clamp is fully open). (Two words)

11. This complication can occur because of an elderly patient's decreased renal function. (Two words)

Down

1. This complication requires culturing the infusion device and the site.

2. This is the most common complication of PCA therapy. (Two words)

5. This is often recognized when a patient needs a higher dose of an opioid analgesic to achieve pain relief.

6. This is the most severe type of hypersensitivity reaction; it can be deadly.

9. A too-rapid injection can cause this type of reaction. (Two words)

In order to treat complications, you've got to be able to spot them first.

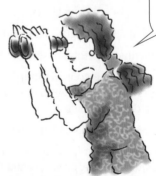

Match point

The Intravenous Nurses Society has developed a classification scale for use in documenting instances of infiltration. Match each degree of infiltration on the left with its accompanying symptom descriptions on the right.

Degree of infiltration

1. 0 _____
2. 1+ _____
3. 2+ _____
4. 3+ _____
5. 4+ _____

Symptom descriptions

A. Blanched skin that's translucent and cool to the touch; gross edema more than 6″ in any direction; mild to moderate pain; possible numbness

B. Blanched skin that's cool to the touch; edema less than 1″ in any direction; possible pain

C. No symptoms

D. Blanched, translucent, tight, leaking, discolored, bruised, or swollen skin; gross edema more than 6″ in any direction; deep, pitting tissue edema; circulatory impairment; moderate to severe pain; infiltration of any amount of blood product, irritant, or vesicant

E. Blanched skin that's cool to the touch; edema 1″ to 6″ in any direction; possible pain

Strikeout

Cross out each of the incorrect statements about phlebitis.

1. Common causes of phlebitis include drugs or solutions that have a high acidity, alkalinity, or osmolarity.

2. Phlebitis can follow any infusion, but it's more common after an I.V. bolus of medication.

3. Phlebitis develops more rapidly in larger veins that are closer to the heart.

4. Typically, phlebitis develops 2 to 3 days after the vein is exposed to the drug or solution.

5. Erythromycin, tetracycline, nafcillin sodium, vancomycin, and amphotericin B are irritating drugs that, when piggybacked, can cause phlebitis.

6. Phlebitis can also result from motion and pressure of the venous access device.

7 Applying ice to the affected area can ease the patient's discomfort.

8. Left untreated, phlebitis can produce exudate at the I.V. site, an elevated white blood cell count, and fever.

If I'm hard, red, tender, and puffy. Watch out—this could be phlebitis!

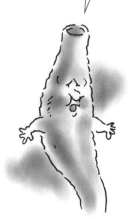

Pep talk

Somehow I can't believe that there are any heights that can't be scaled by a man who knows the secrets of making dreams come true. This special secret, it seems to me, can be summarized in four C s. They are curiosity, confidence, courage, and constancy.

—Walt Disney

■ Jumble gym

Use the clues to help you unscramble words related to the severe local tissue damage incurred when I.V. medication leaks into surrounding tissue. Then use the circled letters to answer the question posed.

Question: Severe local tissue infection can occur with leakage of what kind of blistering agents into the surrounding tissue of an I.V. site?

1. May affect localized wounds or the patient's overall health

Y A D D E L E   N A I L E G H   ◯_ _ _ _◯_ _ _ _ _ _ _◯

2. Another name for cell death

S U I T E S   N O S E S C I R   _ _ _◯_ _ _ _◯_ _ _◯_

3. Medical name for the leakage of caustic drugs into surrounding tissue

A N T I T A R V E X A O S   _ _ _◯_◯_ _ _ _ _

4. Lumps and other abnormalities that can form at affected site

G U M T I D N F I R E S E   _ _◯_ _ _ _ _ _ _ _◯_

5. Surgical removal of affected limb

T A M P I T O N U A   ◯_ _◯_ _◯_ _ _

Answer: _ _ _ _ _ _ _ _   _ _ _ _ _

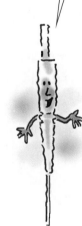

If you're unsure about the patency of an existing I.V. line, you should perform a new venipuncture and establish a new line. I won't hold it against you!

■ Hit or miss

Some of these statements about nursing interventions to prevent or treat extravasation are true; others are false. Mark each with a "T" for "True" or an "F" for "False."

_____ 1. When administering a vesicant drug, the best I.V. sites are the dorsal surface of the patient's hand, the wrist, or the fingers.

_____ 2. You should always start the infusion of a vesicant drug with dextrose 10% in water or half-normal saline solution.

_____ 3. If you suspect extravasation, you should stop the I.V. flow and remove the I.V. line, unless you need the catheter in place to adminsiter the antidote.

_____ 4. You should always administer a vesicant drug by slow I.V. push through a free-flowing I.V. line or by small-volume infusion (50 to 100 ml).

_____ 5. During administration of a vesicant drug, you should observe the site for erythema or infiltration and tell the patient to report any burning, stinging, pain, or sensation of sudden "heat" at the site.

5

Transfusions

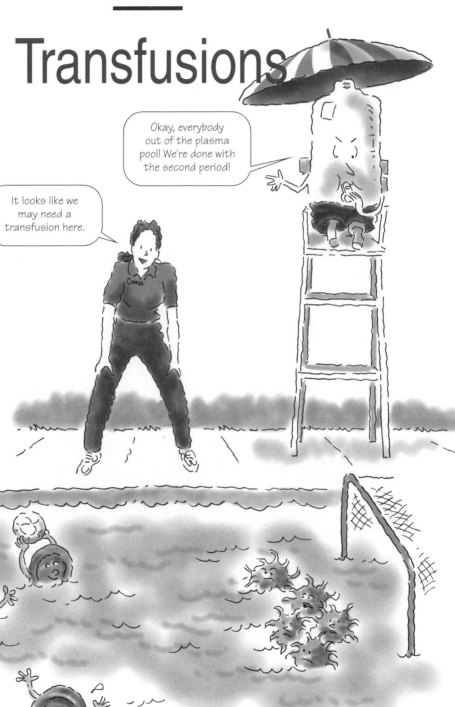

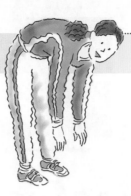

Warm-up

Transfusions review

Purpose

- To restore and maintain blood volume
- To improve the oxygen-carrying capacity of blood
- To replace deficient blood components

Compatibility

- ABO blood type: A, B, AB, O
- Rh blood group: Rh-positive, Rh-negative
- Human leukocyte antigen (HLA) blood group: controls compatibility between transfusion recipients and donors

Transfusion products

Whole blood

- Used to increase blood volume after massive hemorrhage

Leukocyte-poor RBCs

- Used for patients who need red blood cells (RBCs) but who have had a febrile or nonhemolytic reaction in the past

Packed RBCs

- Used to maintain or restore oxygen-carrying capability and capacity

Granulocytes

- Used when granulocytes are low or to fight overwhelming infection

Platelets

- Used to control or prevent bleeding

Plasma and plasma fractions

- Used to correct blood deficiencies, control bleeding tendencies caused by clotting factor deficiencies, and increase circulating blood volume

Transfusion reactions

Hemolytic

- Caused by incompatible blood
- May result in renal failure and shock
- May be life-threatening

Febrile

- Occurs when the patient's anti-HLA antibodies react against the donor's white blood cells (WBCs) or platelets
- Causes flulike symptoms, chest pain, and hypotension

Allergic

- Caused by an allergen present in the transfused blood
- Causes hives, itching, fever, chills, facial swelling, wheezing, and sore throat

Plasma protein incompatibility

- Occurs when blood that contains immunoglobulin A (IgA) proteins is infused into an IgA-deficient recipient who has developed anti-IgA antibodies
- Causes flushing, abdominal pain, chills, fever, hypotension, shock, and cardiac arrest

Bacterial contamination

- Caused by contamination during the collection process
- Causes chills, fever, vomiting, abdominal cramping, diarrhea, shock, and kidney failure

Multiple transfusion reactions

- Hemosiderosis
- Bleeding tendencies
- Increased blood ammonia levels
- Increased oxygen affinity for hemoglobin
- Hypothermia
- Hypocalcemia
- Potassium intoxication

Cross-training

Challenge your memory of blood components and the circulatory system by working the clues to complete this crossword puzzle.

Across

1. Process by which blood forms a solid mass, or clots

4. Another name for RBCs

8. Chronic state of abnormally low RBC levels

11. Name of system identifying individual blood groups

12. Excessive bleeding

13. Life-threatening reaction that occurs when donor and recipient blood types are mismatched

Down

1. Process for determining compatibility of donor and recipient blood

2. Essential element circulated by blood to the body's cells

3. The introduction of whole blood or blood components directly into the bloodstream

5. Another name for platelets

6. One of the benefits of a transfusion is the restoration of this (two words)

7. Inherited antigens usually present on the surface of RBCs (two words)

9. Liquid component of blood

10. Another name for WBCs

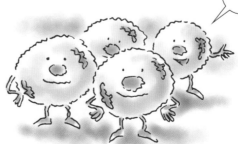

Name tags might be handy in a situation like this. Maybe I'll suggest it at the next ABO group meeting.

■■ Batter's box

Fill in answers from the options below to complete this information about transfusion therapy. Use each option only once.

The _____ is the body's main mover of blood and its components.

₁

The bloodstream carries _____ , nutrients, _____ ,

₂   ₃

and other vital substances to all other tissues and organs of the body. Transfusion

therapy is the introduction of _____ or blood components directly

₄

into the bloodstream. It's used mainly to:

- restore and maintain _____
  ₅

- improve the _____ of blood
  ₆

- replace deficient blood components and improve _____ .
  ₇

> **Options**
>
> A. blood volume
>
> B. circulatory system
>
> C. coagulation
>
> D. hormones
>
> E. oxygen
>
> F. oxygen-carrying capacity
>
> G. whole blood

■■ Power stretch

Stretch your knowledge of transfusion therapy by first unscrambling the words at left to reveal three restorative purposes of a transfusion. Then draw a line from the box to the conditions or diseases on the right that can cause the depletion.

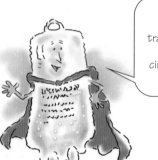

The restorative powers of a blood transfusion are pretty amazing. In some circles, I'm considered a superhero!

DULFI MOLEUV

— — — — —   — — — — — —

EXGONY–RYANGCIR
TAPCYCIA

— — — — — —   -   — — — — — — — —
— — — — — — — —

CLINGOATAOU
PITYCACA

— — — — — — — — — —
— — — — — — — —

A. Acute anemia

B. Bone marrow suppression

C. Burns

D. Carbon monoxide poisoning

E. Coagulopathies

F. Hemorrhage

G. Liver failure

H. Respiratory disorders

I. Sepsis

J. Sickle cell disease

K. Thrombocytopenia

L. Trauma

M. Vitamin K deficiency

■ Strikeout

These statements pertain to transfusion methods and the risks involved. Cross out all of the incorrect statements.

1. Most states permit only licensed registered nurses (not LPNs or vocational nurses) to administer blood and blood components.

2. Transfusions are administered through a peripheral line or a central venous line.

3. Peripheral veins are used for acute transfusions because of their larger diameters and ability to deliver large volumes of blood quickly.

4. A 24-gauge peripheral I.V. catheter is commonly used for transfusions.

5. Because of careful screening and testing, the supply of blood is safer today than it has ever been.

6. Patients receiving transfusions may be at risk for developing hemolytic reactions and exposure to infectious diseases, including human immunodeficiency virus (HIV) and hepatitis.

7. Because transfusion therapy carries few risks and provides great benefits, the patient's consent is unnecessary.

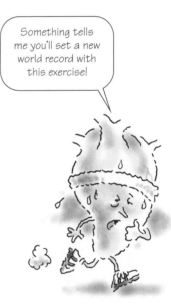

Something tells me you'll set a new world record with this exercise!

■ Mind sprints

Quickly list the four pieces of protective equipment recommended by the Centers for Disease Control and Prevention when transfusing blood or blood products. (This should take 30 seconds or less.)

■ _____

■ _____

■ _____

■ _____

Match point

Blood contains two basic components: cellular elements and plasma. Match each component on the left with its description on the right.

Component

1. Erythrocytes _____
2. Leukocytes _____
3. Plasma proteins _____
4. Serum _____
5. Thrombocytes _____

Description

A. Circulating cells that primarily aid blood clotting; also called *platelets*

B. White cells that defend the body against infectious diseases or foreign particles

C. Clear, watery fluid component found in plasma

D. Transport molecules, enzymes, and regulators that help with cellular processes; include albumin, globulin, and fibrinogen

E. Hemoglobin-carrying cells that are the body's principal means of transporting oxygen from the lungs to cells; also called *red blood cells*

Finish line

Use all of the terms in the box to fill in the pie chart showing the distribution of components making up a patient's total blood volume.

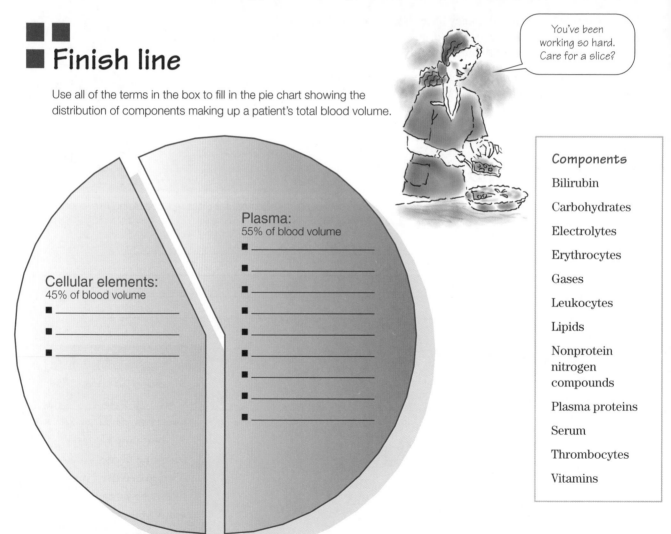

You've been working so hard. Care for a slice?

Plasma:
55% of blood volume
- _____
- _____
- _____
- _____
- _____
- _____
- _____
- _____

Cellular elements:
45% of blood volume
- _____
- _____
- _____

Components

Bilirubin

Carbohydrates

Electrolytes

Erythrocytes

Gases

Leukocytes

Lipids

Nonprotein nitrogen compounds

Plasma proteins

Serum

Thrombocytes

Vitamins

■ Mind sprints

Using the space provided, write down the most important tests used to screen donor and recipient blood for possible incompatibilities. See how many you can list in 2 minutes.

- _____
- _____
- _____
- _____
- _____
- _____

■ Hit or miss

Mark each of these statements about blood compatibility with a "T" for "True" or an "F" for "False."

_____ 1. The most severe type of blood incompatibility is a hemolytic reaction.

_____ 2. A hemolytic reaction destroys WBCs, which help fight off infection.

_____ 3. The four major blood groups are A, B, AB, and O.

_____ 4. An antigen is a substance that can stimulate the formation of an antibody.

_____ 5. Each blood group in the ABO system is named for a specific antibody that is carried on a person's RBCs.

_____ 6. An antibody is an immunoglobulin molecule synthesized in response to a specific antigen.

_____ 7. The ABO system includes two naturally occurring antibodies: anti-AB and anti-O.

_____ 8. The interaction of corresponding antigens and antibodies of the ABO system can cause agglutination (clumping together).

_____ 9. The major antigens, such as those in the ABO system, develop shortly after birth.

_____ 10. Blood transfusions can introduce other antigens and antibodies into the body; most are harmless but could cause a transfusion reaction.

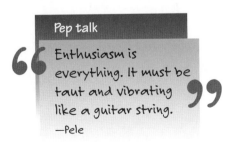

Pep talk

" Enthusiasm is everything. It must be taut and vibrating like a guitar string. "
—Pele

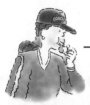

Coaching session
Blood type compatibility

This chart shows blood groups, antibodies present in plasma, and compatible blood types for donating and receiving blood.

Blood group	Antibodies	Can donate to	Can receive from
O	Anti-A, anti-B	O, A, B, AB	O
A	Anti-B	A, AB	A, O
B	Anti-A	B, AB	B, O
AB	Neither anti-A nor anti-B	AB	AB, A, B, O

■ Jumble gym

Use the clues to help you unscramble the words related to blood compatibility. Then use the circled letters to answer the question posed.

> Although blood is thicker than water, unfortunately not everyone is compatible.

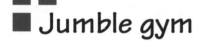

Question: What type of reaction occurs when donor and recipient blood types are mismatched?

1. Person with type O blood

L E A N S V U I R   O B O D L   D R O O N

_ _◯_ _ _ _ _ _   _ _ _◯_   _ _ _ _ _

2. Person lacking anti-A and anti-B antigens

A N E R S L V U I   L O B D O   P I N E T R I E C

_ _ _ _ _ _ _ _ _   _◯_ _ _   _ _ _ _ _ _ _◯_ _

3. Having a high capacity for initiating the body's immune response

G E M I N I N M C O U   _ _◯_ _ _ _ _ _ _◯

4. Proteins found on the surface of cells that are essential to immunity

H A N U M   T O C K L U E Y E   E T S N I N G A

◯_ _ _ _   _ _ _ _ _ _◯_ _   _ _◯_ _ _ _

Answer: _ _ _ _ _ _ _ _ _ _

■■ ■ Strikeout

These statements pertain to Rh blood groups. Cross out all of the incorrect statements.

1. D, or *D factor*, is the most important Rh antigen in the Rh system.

2. The presence or absence of D is one factor that determines whether a person has Rh-positive or Rh-negative blood.

3. Rh-negative blood contains a variant of the D antigen or *D factor*.

4. A person with Rh-negative blood who receives Rh-positive blood will gradually develop anti-Rh antibodies.

5. A serious hemolytic reaction typically follows the first exposure to Rh-positive blood in a person who is Rh-negative.

6. A person with Rh-positive blood doesn't carry anti-Rh antibodies because they would destroy his own RBCs.

7. Most people in the United States have Rh-negative blood.

8. There are two ways that Rh-positive blood can get into Rh-negative blood: by transfusion or during pregnancy in which the fetus has Rh-positive blood.

■■ ■ You make the call

Using the space provided, briefly explain the significance of this blood-grouping combination.

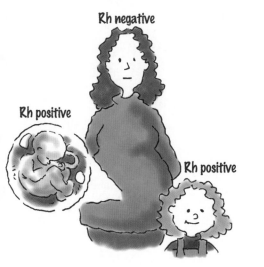

Rh negative

Rh positive

Rh positive

Circuit training

Hemolytic disease of the newborn may occur if Rh immune globulin hasn't been properly administered to an Rh-negative mother who carries and delivers her second Rh-positive fetus. Draw arrows between the boxes to show the order in which the disease progresses.

> During second pregnancy with Rh-positive fetus, mother's anti-Rh antibodies attack fetus, destroying fetal RBCs (hemolysis).

> Fetus produces new RBCs to compensate, but rate of hemolysis escalates, causing the release of bilirubin (red cell component).

> Rh-negative mother becomes sensitized to Rh-positive fetal blood factors during first pregnancy with Rh-positive fetus.

> Fetus's liver can't properly process and excrete bilirubin.

> Fetus is born with jaundice, other liver problems, and possibly brain damage (severity of symptoms depends on rate of hemolysis).

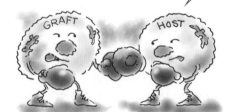

I hope this turns out to be a close HLA match. I don't think I can go another round!

Batter's box

Test your knowledge of the HLA system by filling in the missing information using answers from these options.

Essential to the body's _____ 1 _____ , HLAs are part of the

_____ 2 _____ . This system is responsible for _____ 3 _____ success or

rejection and may play a role in host defense against _____ 4 _____ . It may also

play a role in the triggering of a fatal _____ 5 _____ when WBCs or platelets fail

to multiply after being transfused. Generally, the closer the HLA match between donor

and recipient, the less likely the tissue or organ will be _____ 6 _____ .

HLA testing benefits patients receiving _____ 7 _____ , multiple, or frequent

transfusions. HLA evaluation is also conducted for patients who:

- will receive _____ 8 _____ and _____ 9 _____ transfusions

- will undergo organ or _____ 10 _____ transplant

- have severe or _____ 11 _____ febrile transfusion reactions.

Options

A. cancer

B. graft

C. immune reaction

D. immunity

E. histocompatibility system

F. massive

G. platelet

H. refractory

I. rejected

J. tissue

K. WBC

Power stretch

Stretch your knowledge of transfusions by first unscrambling the words at left to reveal two types of transfused blood. Then draw a line from each type of blood to its specific descriptors at right.

GALOUTOOUS

— — — — — — — — — —

OLOUGSHOOM

— — — — — — — — — —

A. Uses blood collected from a donor

B. Reduces the risks normally associated with transfusions

C. Undergoes rigorous screening and testing to ensure quality

D. Is usually collected and stored shortly before procedure; may be frozen and stored for future need

E. Uses blood collected from the recipient himself

Strikeout

Cross out all of the incorrect statements that pertain to eligibility requirements for donating blood.

1. Donors must be at least 21 and weigh at least 132 lb (60 kg) to give blood.

2. Those with acquired immunodeficiency syndrome (AIDS) can donate blood as long as they are presently taking three HIV drugs and strictly adhere to their medication regimen.

3. Those with hemophilia or who have received clotting factor concentrations can't donate blood.

4. The minimum time between donations is 56 days.

5. Those who have received tattoos within the past 5 years can't donate blood.

6. Anyone who has spent a total of 3 months in the United Kingdom since January 1980 can't donate blood.

7. To donate blood, women must have a hemoglobin level of at least 12.5 g/dl; men, a level of at least 13.5 g/dl.

8. Anyone who has ever used illegal I.V. drugs is ineligible to donate blood.

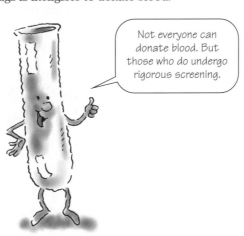

Not everyone can donate blood. But those who do undergo rigorous screening.

Memory jogger

FYI: The most common cause of a severe transfusion reaction is receiving the wrong blood. So, before administering any blood or blood product, always remember to **CVI**:

C: _____

V: _____

I: _____

■ Power stretch

Stretch your knowledge of transfusions by first unscrambling the words at left to reveal commonly transfused blood components. Then draw a line from each component to its nursing considerations and ABO and Rh compatibility requirements on the right. (Note: Each component will have more than one nursing consideration and ABO and Rh compatibility requirement.)

LOWHE OBLOD

— — — — —   — — — — —

CADEPK EDR
BOLDO LESCL

— — — — — —   — — —

— — — — —   — — — — —

TELLAPETS

— — — — — — — — —

RHFSE ONRFZE
PMASAL

— — — — —   — — — — — —

— — — — — —

A. Type A receives Type A or O, type B receives Type B or O, type AB receives type A, AB, B, or O, and type O receives type O.

B. ABO compatibility is required.

C. Use a filtered component drip administration set for this type of infusion.

D. Closely monitor patient's volume status during administration for risk of volume overload.

E. This should be ABO compatible whenever possible.

F. Monitor patient for signs and symptoms of hypocalcemia because the citric acid in this component may bind to calcium.

G. An infusion of this type isn't appropriate for anemias treatable by nutritional or drug therapies.

H. Keep in mind that this is seldom administered.

Pep talk

" Life can be wildly tragic at times, and I've had my share. But whatever happens to you, you have to keep a slightly comic attitude. In the final analysis, you have got not to forget to laugh. "
—Katharine Hepburn

■ Hit or miss

Mark each of these statements about transfused blood components with a "T" for "True" or an "F" for "False."

_____ 1. Packed RBCs consist of blood from which 80% of the RBCs have been removed.

_____ 2. If your patient is receiving whole blood or packed RBCs, you should send for the blood at least 8 hours before it's needed so that it has time to acclimate to room temperature.

_____ 3. Whole blood transfusions are used treat active bleeding with signs and symptoms of hypovolemia.

_____ 4. Packed RBCs are commonly ordered to replace RBCs lost because of GI bleeding, dysmenorrhea, surgery, trauma, or chemotherapy.

_____ 5. Granulocytes (granule-containing leukocytes) are used to control bleeding.

_____ 6. Platelet transfusions aren't usually indicated for conditions of accelerated platelet destruction, such as idiopathic thrombocytopenic purpura or drug-induced thrombocytopenia.

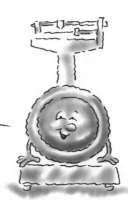

> Did you know that a unit of packed RBCs takes up less volume than whole blood, yet it has the same mass? Pretty heavy stuff!

■ Boxing match

Several methods are used to remove leukocytes from blood. Use the syllables in the boxes to answer clues pertaining to each method. The number of syllables is shown in parentheses. Use each syllable only once.

A	AL	CELL	CEN	CYTE	FIL	FUGE
GENTS	I	ING	KO	LEU	MEN	MOV
RE	SED	TAR	TER	TRI	WASH	Y

1. Uses fibers to trap and separate WBCs

(8) _ _ _ _ _ _ _ _ _ _ _ _ _ _

_ _ _ _ _ _

2. Expensive, yet most ineffective, process that uses special solutions to remove WBCs; also removes about 99% of the plasma

(3) _ _ _ _ _ _ _ _ _ _

3. Spinning device that can be used with filtration and special agents to separate WBCs

(3) _ _ _ _ _ _ _ _ _ _

4. Dextran and hydroxyethyl starch, for example

(7) _ _ _ _ _ _ _ _ _ _ _ _ _ _ _ _

■ Gear up!

Check off the pieces of equipment you might need for a transfusion.

☐ Blood component to be transfused
☐ Blood warmer
☐ Dextrose 5% in water
☐ Foley catheter
☐ Gloves
☐ Goggles
☐ Gown
☐ Infusion pump
☐ In-line or add-on filter
☐ I.V. pole
☐ Mask
☐ N.G. tube
☐ Normal saline solution
☐ Pressure cuff
☐ Sphygmomanometer
☐ Venipuncture equipment
☐ Warfarin

A blood warmer may be ordered to prevent hypothermia and its ensuing arrhythmias, which can occur when administering large volumes of blood quickly.

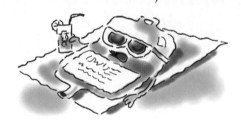

■ Match point

Various types of filters can be used during the transfusion process. Match the description on the right with the type of filter on the left.

Type of filter

1. Standard blood filter _____
2. Microaggregate filter _____
3. Leukocyte reduction filter _____

Description

A. Removes small particles (20- to 40-microns), such as degenerating platelets and fibrin strands, from blood

B. Traps blood particles that are 170 microns or larger

C. Screens out WBCs from transfused whole blood, packed RBCs, or platelets

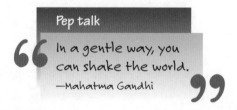

■■
■ Mind sprints

In 30 seconds or less, list four reasons to return a blood bag to the blood bank upon inspecting it before starting an infusion.

■ _____

■ _____

■ _____

■ _____

■■
■ Starting lineup

Show that you know the proper way to prepare a Y-type transfusion setup by putting these steps in the correct order.

Hang both bags on the I.V. pole.	
Attach the blood administration set to the venous access device using a needleless connection, and flush it with the normal saline solution.	
Remove the adapter cover at the tip of the blood administration set, open the main flow clamp, and prime the tubing with normal saline solution; close the clamp and recap the adapter.	
Insert the spike of the line you're using for the normal saline solution into the saline solution bag.	
Gather a Y-type blood administration set, an I.V. pole, and a venous access device.	
Close all the clamps on the I.V. administration set.	
Open the port on the blood bag, and insert the spike of the line you're using to administer the blood or blood component into the port.	
Open the clamp on the line of normal saline solution, and squeeze the drip chamber until it's half full of normal saline solution.	

■ Finish line

Does your blood type compatibility knowledge measure up? Fill in the missing values to find out.

Blood group	Compatible RBCs
Recipient	
O	_____ 1
A	_____ 2
B	B, O
AB	_____ 3
Donor	
O	O, A, B, AB
A	_____ 4
B	B, AB
AB	_____ 5

■ Strikeout

These statements pertain to the transfusion process. Cross out all of the incorrect statements.

1. Priming the filter and I.V. tubing with normal saline solution reduces the risk of microclots forming in the tubing during an infusion.

2. When administering whole blood or WBCs, you should invert the bag several times during the procedure to mix the cells, and gently agitate the bag to prevent the cells from settling.

3. Generally, a transfusion is run at a fast flow rate of 85 gtt/minute for the first 10 to 30 minutes.

4. A unit of RBCs is typically given over a period of 1 to 4 hours.

5. Platelets and coagulation factors may be given more slowly than RBCs and granulocytes.

6. A transfusion shouldn't take more than 8 hours.

7. Any unused blood following a transfusion can be resealed and stored on the nursing unit for future emergency use.

8. It's extremely important to monitor the patient's vital signs every 10 minutes throughout the transfusion.

9. You should always have sterile normal saline solution set up as a primary line along with the transfusion in case a transfusion reaction occurs.

Remember that the risk of contamination and sepsis increases 4 hours after a transfusion begins, so watch the time closely.

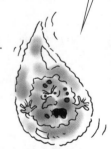

■■
■ Mind sprints

Quickly list six common signs and symptoms of a hemolytic
transfusion reaction that require you to immediately stop a transfusion.
Then list two additional symptoms that typically accompany an anaphylactic
reaction. See if you can list all eight symptoms in 1 minute.

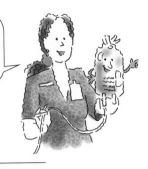

> Keep sterile saline
> solution on standby during
> a transfusion. You may
> need it in a hurry!

- _____
- _____
- _____
- _____
- _____
- _____
- _____
- _____

■■
■ Starting lineup

Transfusion reactions require prompt action. Show that you know what action to take if the patient shows any sign of a
transfusion reaction by putting these steps in the correct order.

Notify the practitioner.	
Check and record the patient's vital signs.	
Reestablish the normal saline infusion (if using a straight-line infusion); if using a Y-set, use a new bag of saline solution and tubing.	
Monitor the patient throughout the entire transfusion.	
Quickly clamp the blood infusion line to stop the transfusion; don't dispose of the blood bag.	
Continue to observe the patient; if no additional signs of a reaction appear within 15 minutes, adjust the flow clamp to achieve the ordered infusion rate, as ordered.	

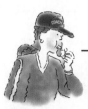

Coaching session
Five transfusion don'ts

 Don't add medications to the blood bag.

Don't give blood products without first checking the order against the blood bag—the only way to tell if the request form has been stamped with the wrong name.

Don't transfuse the blood product if you discover a discrepancy in the blood number, blood slip type, or patient identification number.

Don't piggyback blood into the port of an existing infusion set.

Don't hesitate to stop the transfusion if your patient has changes in vital signs or shows any evidence of a transfusion reaction.

■ You make the call

Identify the device shown in the illustration here, and briefly explain in the spaces provided why it's used.

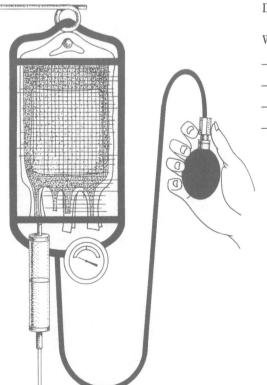

Device: _____

Why it's used: _____

_____

_____

_____

_____

■■ ■ Starting lineup

Show that you understand the proper procedure for using a pressure cuff during rapid blood administration by putting these steps in the correct sequence.

Prepare the patient, and set up the equipment as you would with a straight-line blood administration set.

Hang the pressure cuff and blood bag on the I.V. pole; open the flow clamp on the tubing.

Connect the tubing to the catheter hub.

Prime the filter and tubing with normal saline solution to remove all air from the administration set.

Set the flow rate by turning the screw clamp on the pressure cuff counterclockwise; compress the pressure bulb of the cuff to inflate the bag to the desired flow rate. Then turn the screw clamp clockwise to maintain this constant rate.

Insert your hand into the top of the pressure cuff sleeve, and pull the blood bag through the center opening; hang the blood bag loop on the hook provided with the sleeve.

> As the blood bag empties, the pressure decreases, so check the flow rate regularly and adjust the pressure cuff as necessary to maintain a consistent rate.

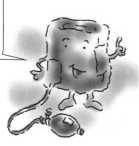

■■ ■ Hit or miss

Mark each statement about the transfusion procedure with a "T" for "True" or an "F" for "False."

_____ 1. Most hemolytic reactions occur during the first 30 minutes of a transfusion.

_____ 2. Increasing the pressure of a blood transfusion with a pressure cuff slows the speed at which complications develop.

_____ 3. As long as the pressure cuff maintains equal, constant pressure throughout the transfusion, the pressure can be set at the highest maximum setting.

_____ 4. After the transfusion is complete, you should flush the tubing with an adequate amount of normal saline solution according to the patient's condition.

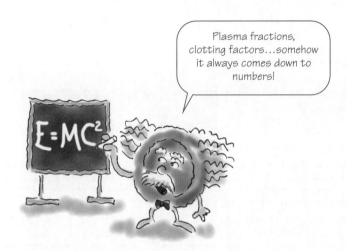

Plasma fractions, clotting factors...somehow it always comes down to numbers!

■ Batter's box

Complete this information about blood components by filling in answers from the options below. Use each option only once.

Plasma and _____ comprise the anticoagulated clear portion of blood

<u>1</u>

that has been run through a _____ . These blood components make up

<u>2</u>

about 55% of total blood volume and are used to:

- correct blood deficiencies such as a low _____

  <u>3</u>

- control bleeding tendencies that result from _____ deficiencies

  <u>4</u>

- increase the patient's _____ .

  <u>5</u>

  Plasma substitutes may be used to maintain blood volume in an emergency, such

as _____ and shock. Plasma substitutes lack _____ and

<u>6</u>   <u>7</u>

coagulation properties, but using them allows for time to get the patient's blood

typed and _____ .

<u>8</u>

Options

A. acute hemorrhage

B. centrifuge

C. circulating blood volume

D. clotting factor

E. crossmatched

F. oxygen-carrying

G. plasma fractions

H. platelet count

Power stretch

Stretch your knowledge of blood components once again by first unscrambling the words at left to reveal four blood components. Then draw a line from each box to the nursing considerations and indications on the right. (Note: Each component will have more than one nursing consideration and indication.)

REOTCCYPIRTPAEI

_ _ _ _ _ _ _ _ _ _ _ _ _ _ _

OCFATR IVII

_ _ _ _ _ _   _ _ _ _

AIULBNM

_ _ _ _ _ _ _

MMENUI OINUGLLB

_ _ _ _ _ _   _ _ _ _ _ _ _ _

A. Administer this cautiously in patients with cardiac and pulmonary disease because heart failure may result from volume overload.

B. Add normal saline solution to each bag of this, as necessary, to facilitate transfusion.

C. This is indicated for volume loss due to burns, trauma, surgery, or infection.

D. Administer this by I.V. injection using a filter needle or use the administration set supplied by the manufacturer.

E. This is indicated for neurologic disorders.

F. This is indicated for significant factor XIII deficiency.

G. Reconstitute the lyophilized powder with normal saline solution injection, 5% dextrose, or sterile water.

H. This is indicated for von Willebrand's disease.

Pep talk

" In order to excel, you must be completely dedicated to your chosen sport. You must also be prepared to work hard and be willing to accept destructive criticism. Without 100 percent dedication, you won't be able to do this. "

—Willie Mays

■ Train your brain

Sound out each group of pictures and symbols to reveal important information about blood components and transfusions.

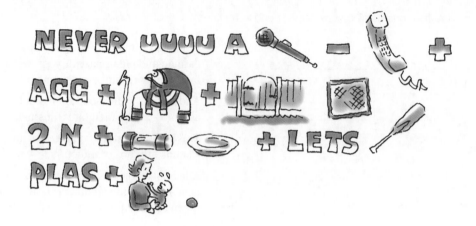

■ Match point

Plasma and plasma products are used to treat a variety of specific disorders. Match the plasma products on the left with the disorders on the right.

Plasma products

1. Fresh frozen plasma _____

2. Albumin _____

3. Factor VIII concentrate _____

Disorders

A. Hemophilia A; bleeding; coagulation factor deficiency

B. Postsurgical hemorrhage or shock; factor deficiencies resulting from hepatic disease or other causes

C. Volume loss from burns, trauma, surgery, or infections; hypoproteinemia (with or without edema)

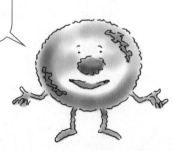

Depending on the circumstances, in an emergency you may be able to give a synthetic volume expander, such as dextran in saline solution, or a natural volume expander, such as plasma protein fraction and albumin.

■ Strikeout

These statements pertain to plasma products. Cross out any incorrect statements.

1. Using a microaggregate filter to transfuse plasma products could remove essential components.
2. You should always use a 24- to 26-gauge venous access device to transfuse fresh frozen plasma in an emergency.
3. Large-volume transfusions of fresh frozen plasma may require correction for hypercalcemia.
4. Cross-typing is always necessary when administering albumin.
5. Albumin is contraindicated as an expander in severe anemia.
6. You should always administer factor VIII concentrate slowly to prevent a hemolytic reaction.
7. The risk of hepatitis is high when administering prothrombin complex to a patient.
8. Cryoprecipitate and factor VIII are essentially the same.
9. Factor IX, or *antihemophilic factor*, is commonly used to treat hemophilia A.
10. Plasma products typically have a cloudy or turbid appearance.

■ Batter's box

Use answers from the options below to fill in this information about specialized transfusion methods.

Specialized methods for administering blood include:

- _____ , the process of collecting, filtering, and reinfusing the patient's

    own blood; and

- _____ , the process of collecting and removing specific blood

    components and then returning the remaining components to the donor.

    Many patients prefer autotransfusion because it eliminates the risk of

_____ . Blood can be collected beginning 4 to 6 weeks before

_____ ; units are then labeled and stored until needed. Blood collected

during surgery is treated with an _____ and collected in a sterile container

fitted with a _____ . The blood is _____ as whole blood or

processed before infusion. Any _____ blood can't be stored because the

filtering and processing can't remove _____ completely.

> **Options**
> A. anticoagulant
> B. autotransfusion
> C. bacteria
> D. filter
> E. hemapheresis
> F. infectious disease
> G. reinfused
> H. salvaged
> I. surgery

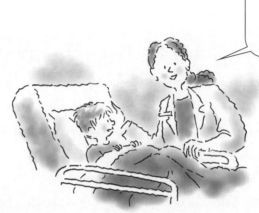

Remember, children aren't little adults. They have specific I.V. needs.

In the ballpark

Transfusions in children differ significantly from transfusions in adults. Show that you know the differences by circling the correct answer in each column.

	Adults			Children		
Total blood volume	2.5 L	5 L	8 L	75 ml/kg	100 ml/kg	125 ml/kg
Prepared blood units	½ unit	1 unit	2 units	½ unit	1 unit	2 units
Catheter size	20 gauge	24 gauge	28 gauge	18 gauge	20 gauge	24 gauge

Hit or miss

Mark each statement about the special needs of pediatric and elderly patients with a "T" for "True" or an "F" for "False."

_____ 1. Usually, children receive 5% to 10% of the total transfusion in the first 15 minutes of therapy.

_____ 2. To maintain the correct flow rate in children, you should use an electronic infusion device.

_____ 3. The proportion of blood volume to body weight increases as a child ages.

_____ 4. As long as the parents have been informed, it's unnecessary to explain the transfusion procedure to an older child.

_____ 5. In massive hemorrhage and shock, the indications for blood component transfusion in children tend to be similar to those in adults.

_____ 6. An elderly patient with preexisting heart disease should be able to tolerate receiving a rapid transfusion of an entire unit of blood without any adverse effects.

_____ 7. Elderly patients have a lower risk of delayed or severe transfusion reactions than younger patients do.

_____ 8. Elderly patients are usually more resistant than younger patients to transfusion-related infections.

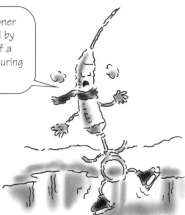

Expect the practitioner to order ice followed by warm compresses if a hematoma develops during a transfusion.

Starting lineup

A hematoma can develop at the I.V. site during a transfusion. Show that you know how to handle the situation by putting these steps in the correct order.

Notify the practitioner.	
Remove the catheter.	
Prepare to ice the site. (The site is usually iced for 24 hours, then warm compresses are applied.)	
Document your observations and actions.	
Cap the tubing with a new needleless connection.	
Stop the infusion.	
Promote reabsorption of the hematoma by having the patient gently exercise the affected limb.	

Strikeout

These statements pertain to the possible nursing actions you can take when a transfusion suddenly stops. Cross out all of the incorrect nursing actions.

1. Check that the container is at least 12″ (30.5 cm) above the level of the I.V. site.

2. Make sure the flow clamp is open.

3. Make sure the blood completely covers the filter. If it doesn't, squeeze the drip chamber until it does.

4. Check to see if any blood cells have settled to the bottom of the bag; if so, the blood must be replaced.

5. If using a Y-type blood administration set, close the flow clamp to the patient and lower the blood bag; open the clamp to the normal saline solution line, and allow it to flow into the blood bag; then rehang the bag, open the flow clamp to the patient, and reset the flow rate.

■■
■ Jumble gym

Use the clues to help you unscramble words related to reactions that can occur from any transfusion. Then use the circled letters to answer the question posed.

Question: What type of drug, besides an antihistamine, is typically ordered to treat a nonhemolytic febrile reaction?

1. Life-threatening reaction that occurs from incompatible blood

C A T E U   Y O H I M T C L E   T E A R C O I N

_ _ _ (_) _   _ _ _ _ _ (_) _ _   _ _ (_) _ _ _ _

2. Characterized by a temperature increase of 1.8° F (1° C); usually results from patient's anti-HLA antibodies reacting against antigens on the donor's white blood cells or platelets

B I L F E R E   C A R T O E N I   _ _ _ _ (_) _ _   _ _ _ _ _ _ _ _ _

3. Second most common reaction; occurs because of an allergen in the transfused blood

R E A L G I L C   O R A C N I T E

_ _ _ (_) _ _ _   _ _ _ _ (_) _ _ _

4. Results when blood containing immunoglobulin A (IgA) is infused into an IgA-deficient recipient who has developed ant-IgA antibodies

S A M P A L   T O N R I P E   P L I N I M O T I B A T Y I C

(_) _ _ _ _ _   _ _ _ _ _ _ _   _ (_) _ _ _ _ _ _ _ _ (_) _ _ _

5. Caused by endotoxins that contaminate blood during the blood collection or storage process

L A T E A R B I C   T I N T M A I N C A N O O

_ _ _ (_) _ _ _ _   (_) _ _ _ _ _ _ _ _ _ _ _ _ _

Answer: _ _ _ _ _ _ _ _ _ _ _

■■
■ Mind sprints

As quickly as you can, list 10 signs and symptoms of a nonhemolytic febrile reaction. See if you can list all 10 in 2 minutes or less.

■ _____   ■ _____
■ _____   ■ _____
■ _____   ■ _____
■ _____   ■ _____
■ _____   ■ _____

■■
■ Match point

It's important to learn to recognize signs and symptoms of transfusion reactions because such reactions can be fatal if treatment isn't prompt. Match the transfusion reaction on the left with it's signs and symptoms on the right.

Transfusion reaction

1. Allergic reaction _____

2. Plasma protein incompatibility _____

3. Bacterial contamination _____

4. Hemolytic reaction _____

Signs and symptoms

A. Chills, fever, vomiting, abdominal cramping, diarrhea, shock, kidney failure

B. Itching, hives, fever, chills, facial swelling, wheezing, throat swelling

C. Flushing and urticaria, abdominal pain, fever, dyspnea and wheezing, hypotension, shock, cardiac arrest

D. Chest pain, dyspnea, facial flushing, fever, chills, hypotension, flank pain, burning along the vein receiving blood, shock, renal failure

> Protect your patient from transfusion reactions by taking necessary precautions and remaining vigilant during the infusion.

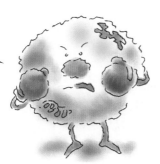

■■
■ Hit or miss

Mark each statement about transfusion reactions with a "T" for "True" or an "F" for "False."

_____ 1. Febrile reactions are relatively rare, occurring in only about 1% of all transfusions.

_____ 2. An acute hemolytic reaction isn't considered life-threatening because the symptoms aren't serious and they tend to develop slowly.

_____ 3. An allergic reaction can progress to an anaphylactic reaction up to 1 hour after infusion.

_____ 4. Severe anaphylactic reactions produce bronchospasm, dyspnea, pulmonary edema, and hypotension.

_____ 5. The bacterial infections associated with transfusion are most commonly caused by endotoxins produced by gram-positive bacteria.

_____ 6. To prevent a febrile reaction, patients may be premedicated with an antipyretic, an antihistamine, and possibly a steroid.

_____ 7. Any blood bag with gas, clots, or a dark purple color shouldn't be used because it may be a sign of plasma protein incompatibility.

Boxing match

Identify commonly used treatments for transfusion reactions by filling in answers to the clues using all the syllables in the boxes below. The number of syllables for each answer appears in parentheses. Use each syllable only once.

AN	AN	AN	BI	BROAD	DI	EP	HIS
I	IC	MINE	NEPH	O	OT	PRES	PY
RE	RE	RINE	SOR	SPEC	TA	TI	TI
TI	TIC	TIC	TRUM	U	VAS		

1. Also called *adrenaline*; used for emergency circulatory response to hemolytic and allergic reactions

   (4) _ _ _ _ _ _ _ _ _ _ _

2. Drug that aids in the bodily excretion of urine; helps in hemolytic reactions and circulatory overload

   (4) _ _ _ _ _ _ _ _

3. Vasoconstrictor that aids in increasing blood pressure in the treatment of shock

   (4) _ _ _ _ _ _ _ _ _ _

4. Fever-fighting agent used to treat febrile reactions

   (5) _ _ _ _ _ _ _ _ _ _ _

5. Drug that reduces the effects of chemicals released in response to an allergen

   (5) _ _ _ _ _ _ _ _ _ _ _ _ _

6. Drug that helps fight a wide range of bacteria

   (8) _ _ _ _ _ - _ _ _ _ _ _ _ _
   _ _ _ _ _ _ _ _

NCLEX reps

Test your knowledge of transfusion reactions with this NCLEX-style question.

Question: A nurse is administering a blood transfusion to a client with sickle cell anemia. Which assessment findings would indicate that the client is having a transfusion reaction?

1. Diaphoresis and hot flashes
2. Urticaria, flushing, and wheezing
3. Fever, urticaria, and red raised rash
4. Fever, disorientation, and abdominal pain

> If you can't think of the correct term, don't have an "over-reaction." just skip over the word and come back to it later!

Cross-training

Test your knowledge of transfusion reactions with this crossword puzzle.

Across

4. Results from citrate toxicity when blood is transfused too rapidly

8. Type of contamination associated with growth of microorganisms

9. Antihistamines may be given to prevent or treat this type of reaction

12. Fever-reducing agent given to combat febrile reactions

13. May result from a low platelet count; includes abnormal bleeding, oozing from cuts (Two words)

14. Hemoglobin saturation shift noted on oxyhemoglobin dissociation curve (Two words)

Down

1. Blood levels of this may be high with transfusion of stored blood

2. May occur with rapid transfusion of cold blood

3. Marked by temperature increase from the transfusion and not from disease (Two words)

5. To prevent, transfuse blood slowly and don't exceed 2 units in 4 hours (Two words)

6. Accumulation of iron-containing pigment that occurs in patients receiving many transfusions

7. Incompatibility that may be prevented by transfusing only immunoglobulin A-deficient blood or well-washed RBCs (Two words)

10. Toxic levels of this cation may result when RBCs leak into the plasma of stored blood

11. Type of reaction resulting from blood incompatibility or improper storage of blood

■ Hit or miss

Mark each statement about transfusions and infectious disease with a "T" for "True" and an "F" for "False."

_____ 1. Because of the latest blood testing and screening methods, it's virtually impossible to transmit an infectious disease during a transfusion.

_____ 2. Signs and symptoms of infectious diseases are always apparent within a few days after transmittal.

_____ 3. Most posttransfusion cases of hepatitis involve the transmission of hepatitis B.

_____ 4. The test that detects hepatitis C yields highly accurate results; therefore, any cases of posttransfusion hepatitis C can only occur because of failure to screen for the disease.

_____ 5. HIV screening determines the presence of antibodies and antigens to HIV.

_____ 6. False-negative results can occur with HIV screening, particularly during the incubation period (about 6 to 12 weeks after exposure).

_____ 7. Screening for cytomegalovirus (CMV) is rarely done because of its expense.

_____ 8. Receiving blood with CMV is especially dangerous for an immunosuppressed, seronegative patient.

_____ 9. Because syphilis has been virtually eradicated, only potential donors who were exposed to the disease within the past 10 years are routinely tested.

_____ 10. Blood warmers are used as an added precaution to kill off any syphilis organisms that go undetected.

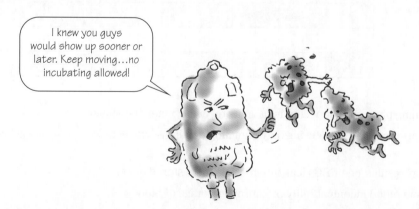

6

Chemotherapy infusions

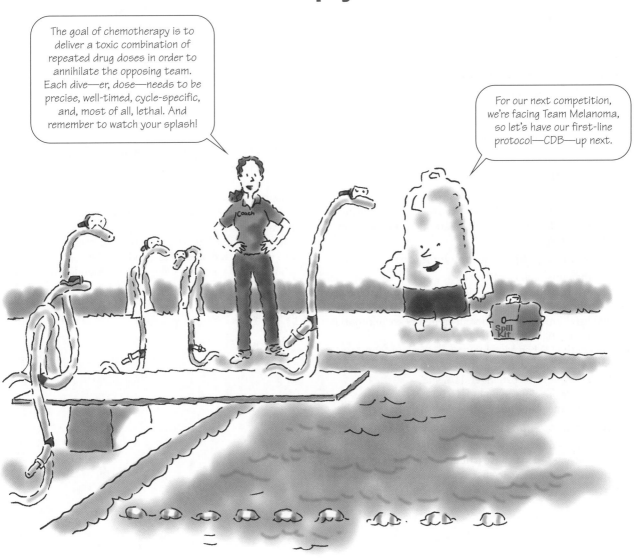

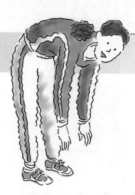

Chemotherapy infusions review

Chemotherapy infusion

- Usually calls for more than one drug to target different cancer cell phases
- Works best when the most effective drug is chosen as the first line
- Requires three treatment cycles for most patients

Chemotherapeutic drugs

- Categorized according to their action and how they interfere with cell production
- May be cycle-specific (act during specific phases of a cell cycle) or cycle-nonspecific (act on reproducing and resting cells)

Immunotherapy

- Enhances the body's ability to destroy cancer cells
- Involves administration of monoclonal antibodies, which target tumor cells, or immunomodulatory cytokines, which affect immune response

Administering chemotherapy infusions

- Perform a preadministration check.
- Prepare chemotherapeutic drugs using appropriate protective measures.
- Establish I.V. access. (Peripheral catheters are appropriate; use smallest gauge possible.)
- Connect the I.V. bag containing normal saline solution to the I.V. catheter before giving the drug.
- Closely monitor the patient and I.V. site.
- Properly dispose of equipment.
- Document the procedure.

Chemotherapeutic drugs and tissue damage

- Vesicants—cause blisters and severe tissue damage
- Nonvesicants—don't cause irritation or tissue damage
- Irritants—cause a local venous response, with or without a skin reaction

Infusion-site complications

INFILTRATION
- Results from nonvesicant leaking into surrounding tissue
- Causes swelling, blanching, and possible flow-rate change

EXTRAVASATION
- Results from vesicant leaking into surrounding tissue
- Causes swelling, pain, and blanching

VEIN FLARE
- Results from irritant drug
- Causes vein to become red and surrounded by hives

Adverse effects of chemotherapy

- Alopecia (hair loss)—may be minimal or severe
- Anaphylactic reaction—may occur any time during drug administration
- Diarrhea—may lead to weight loss, electrolyte imbalance, and malnutrition
- Myelosuppression—damage to precursors of white blood cells (WBCs), red blood cells, and platelets
- Nausea and vomiting—may be anticipated, acute, or delayed
- Secondary malignancy—usually occurs after use of alkalating agents

◼◼ ◼ Batter's box

Fill in this information about chemotherapy infusions with answers from the options box.

Chemotherapy, _____ , and _____ are the mainstays of cancer
1   2

treatment. Most commonly administered I.V., using peripheral or central veins,

chemotherapy may also be given by the oral, subcutaneous, _____ , I.M.,
3

intra-arterial, and _____ routes.
4

    The benefits of I.V. chemotherapy include the ability to deliver an exact dose of a

_____ drug to suppress rapidly dividing cancer cells. Additional benefits
5

include complete _____ of the drug and _____ distribution of
6   7

the drug throughout the circulation. Unfortunately, although chemotherapy is intended to

control or eliminate _____ cells, it can also damage _____
8   9

cells, attacking all rapidly growing cells regardless of type. Because _____
10

and _____ are rapidly growing cells, chemotherapy patients typically lose
11

their hair and their nails become _____ .
12

    Long-term chemotherapy, which involves frequent _____ , can make veins
13

_____ . Patients may also be at risk for _____ or
14   15

_____ with the use of certain chemotherapeutic drugs.
16

Options
A. absorption
B. brittle
C. cancerous
D. hair
E. healthy
F. intracavitary
G. intrathecal
H. nail follicles
I. phlebitis
J. radiation
K. sclerotic
L. surgery
M. systemic
N. tissue necrosis
O. toxic
P. venipunctures

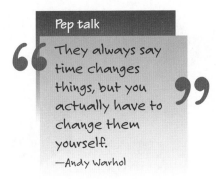

Pep talk

" They always say
time changes
things, but you
actually have to
change them
yourself. "
—Andy Warhol

◼◼
◼ Power stretch

Stretch your knowledge of how chemotherapy works by unscrambling the words at left to reveal two types of drugs that help fight cancerous cells. Then draw a line from the boxes to the corresponding descriptions at right.

C L E L   C L E C Y – E F S C I C I P

_ _ _ _   _ _ _ _ _ _   –
_ _ _ _ _ _ _ _ _ _

L E C L   L Y E C C – P S N I F C O N E I C

_ _ _ _   _ _ _ _ _ _   –
_ _ _ _ _ _ _ _ _ _ _ _ _

A. Are designed to disrupt a specific biochemical process

B. Act on both reproducing and resting cells

C. Have a prolonged action that's independent of the cell cycle

D. Are effective only during specific phases of the cell cycle

E. Allow a fixed percentage of normal and malignant cells to live or die

F. Allow cells in the resting phase to survive

◼◼
◼ Finish line

All cells cycle through five phases. Some chemotherapeutic drugs are active during one or more of the phases, as shown here. Use these clues to identify the specific cell cycle phases.

1. _____
Deoxyribonucleic acid (DNA) synthesis halts. Ribonucleic acid (RNA) and protein synthesis continues in preparation for mitosis.

2. _____
Mitosis occurs. Daughter cells may repeat the cell cycle or enter the G_0 phase.

3. _____
Resting occurs. Some cells will replicate while others will remain inactive.

Because tumor cells are active in various phases of the cell cycle, chemotherapy typically uses more than one drug—this way, each drug can target a different site or take action during a different phase.

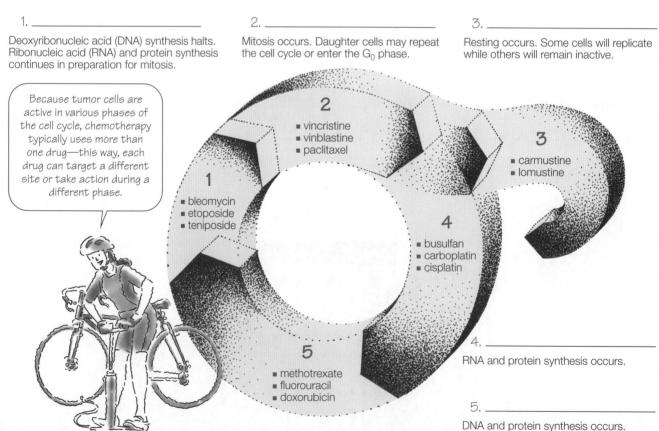

2
■ vincristine
■ vinblastine
■ paclitaxel

3
■ carmustine
■ lomustine

1
■ bleomycin
■ etoposide
■ teniposide

4
■ busulfan
■ carboplatin
■ cisplatin

5
■ methotrexate
■ fluorouracil
■ doxorubicin

4. _____
RNA and protein synthesis occurs.

5. _____
DNA and protein synthesis occurs.

■■
■ Mind sprints

List two reasons why chemotherapeutic drugs are given in combination. (This one requires a little thought. Time yourself, and see if you can list both answers in 2 minutes or less.)

■ _____

■ _____

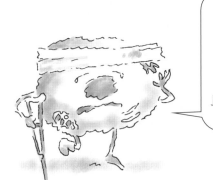

The challenge of chemotherapy is to provide a drug dose large enough to kill the greatest number of cancer cells but small enough to avoid irreversibly damaging normal tissue or causing toxicity. Let's just say I was in the wrong place at the wrong time!

■■
■ Strikeout

These statements pertain to the chemotherapeutic drug selection process. Cross out all of the incorrect statements.

1. Drug selection depends primarily on five things: the patient's age, overall condition, tumor type, allergies or sensitivities, and the stage of cancer.

2. Generally, the drugs chosen for the first round of chemotherapy are the least effective.

3. Second- or third-line chemotherapy drugs may be used depending on the patient's hypersensitivity reactions or the tumor's resistance to first-line drugs.

4. A single course of chemotherapy involves administering one dose of a single drug.

5. Treatment cycles are planned so that normal cells can regenerate.

6. Most patients require six treatment cycles before they show any beneficial response.

7. Chemotherapeutic drugs are commonly given in combinations called _protocols_.

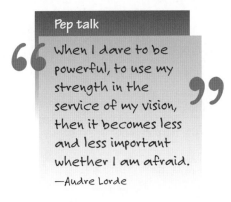

Pep talk

" When I dare to be powerful, to use my strength in the service of my vision, then it becomes less and less important whether I am afraid. "
—Audre Lorde

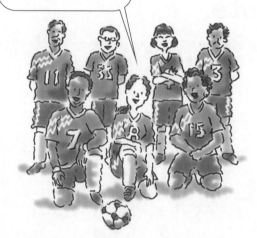

We're all on the same team when it comes to stopping and slowing the growth of cancerous cells!

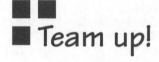

Team up!

Chemotherapeutic drugs are categorized according to their pharmacologic action as well as the way in which they interfere with cell production. Write the drug class name under the appropriate cell-cycle category. Use all of the options listed.

Cell cycle–specific drugs

_____

_____

_____

Cell cycle–nonspecific drugs

_____

_____

_____

_____

_____

Drug classifications
- Alkylating agents
- Antibiotic antineoplastics
- Antimetabolites
- Antineoplastics
- Enzymes
- Miscellaneous
- Nitrosureas
- Plant alkaloids

Boxing match

Use all of the syllables in the boxes below to answer clues about other drugs that inhibit tumor cell growth. The number of syllables for each answer is shown in parentheses. Use each syllable only once.

AN	HOR	HOR	MONES	MONES	ROIDS	STE	TI

1. Normally act as anti-inflammatory agents; make malignant cells vulnerable to damage from cell-specific drugs

(2) __ __ __ __ __ __ __ __ __

2. Alter the environment of cells by affecting the permeability of their membranes

(2) __ __ __ __ __ __ __ __

3. Affect hormone-dependent tumors by inheriting the production of those hormones or neutralizing their effects

(4) __ __ __ __ __ __ __ __ __ __ __ __

Power stretch

Stretch your knowledge by first unscrambling the words at left to reveal eight classes of chemotherapeutic drugs. Then draw a line from each box to the examples and characteristics of each drug class on the right.

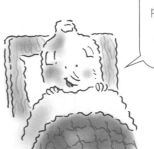

Chemotherapeutic drugs are used to control cancer, cure cancer, or prevent metastasis. They're also used as a palliative measure to help make the patient feel better.

MATEBESTLOANITI

_ _ _ _ _ _ _ _ _ _ _ _ _

NLPAT KIDLALASO

_ _ _ _ _   _ _ _ _ _ _ _ _ _

SMEZYEN

_ _ _ _ _ _ _

TALLYAKING STAGEN

_ _ _ _ _ _ _ _ _ _
_ _ _ _ _ _

OCTINBITAI SPANCINTLEASTOI

_ _ _ _ _ _ _ _ _
_ _ _ _ _ _ _ _ _ _ _ _ _

RESHMOON NAD NOROHME
ITHIRSINOB

_ _ _ _ _ _ _   _ _
_ _ _ _ _ _ _
_ _ _ _ _ _ _ _ _

COLIF IDAC LONGASA

_ _ _ _ _   _ _ _
_ _ _ _ _ _ _

PYOTTICROCVEET GATESN

_ _ _ _ _ _ _ _ _ _ _ _ _ _
_ _ _ _ _ _

A. Antidote for methotrexate toxicity; includes leucovorin

B. Useful only in leukemias; includes asparaginase

C. Interfere with nucleic acid synthesis; attack during S phase of cell cycle; include cytarabine, fluoxuridine, fluorouracil, hydroxyurea, methotrexate, and thioguanine

D. Disrupt DNA replication; include carboplatin, cisplatin, cyclophosphamide, ifosfamide, and thiotepa

E. Protect normal tissue by binding with metabolites of other cytotoxic drugs; include dexrazoxane and mesna

F. Prevent mitotic spindle formation; cycle-specific to M phase; include vinblastine and vincristine

G. Interfere with binding of normal hormones to receptor proteins, manipulate hormone levels, and alter hormone environment; usually palliative, not curative; include androgens (testolactone), antiandrogens (flutamide), antiestrogens (tamoxifen), estrogens (estramustine), gonadotropin (leuprolide), and progestins (megestrol)

H. Bind with DNA to inhibit synthesis of DNA and RNA; include bleomycin, doxorubicin, idarubicin, mitoxantrone, and mitomycin

■ Hit or miss

Mark each of these statements about cancer immunotherapy with a "T" for "True" or an "F" for "False."

_____ 1. Cancer immunotherapy seeks to evoke effective immune response to tumors by altering the way cells grow, mature, and respond to cancer cells.

_____ 2. The drugs used in cancer immunotherapy are called *cellumorphic stimulators* because they enhance the body's ability to destroy cancer cells.

_____ 3. Cancer immunotherapy is unique because it manipulates the body's natural resources instead of introducing toxic substances that aren't selective and can't differentiate between normal or abnormal processes or cells.

_____ 4. The two main classes of immunotherapy drugs used to fight cancer are monoclonal antibodies and immunomodulatory cytokines.

■ Batter's box

Use answers from these options to complete the following information on monoclonal antibodies.

Monoclonal antibodies, which specifically target _____ , are a

form of immunotherapy. Antibodies are _____ produced by

mature _____ or plasma cells in response to

_____ —proteins found on the surface of normal and

abnormal cells. Antibodies recognize specific antigens and bind exclusively

to them; this process is referred to as a _____ . Such binding

causes tumor cell _____ or destruction.

Options
A. antigens
B. B cells
C. immunoglobulins
D. inactivation
E. lock-and-key mechanism
F. tumor cells

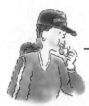

Coaching session
Fighting cancer with monoclonal antibodies

Three monoclonal antibodies have been approved by the Food and Drug Administration for cancer therapy:
• rituximab (Rituxan)—used specifically for relapsed or refractory low-grade Hodgkin's disease and non-Hodgkin's lymphoma
• trastuzumab (Herceptin)—effective against metastatic breast cancer; may be used as a first-line treatment with other chemotherapeutic agents or as a second-line single agent
• bevacizumab (Avastin)—used to treat metastatic colon cancer; first monoclonal antibody that prevents formation of new blood vessels so that tumor cells don't receive blood, oxygen, and other nutrients needed for growth.

Jumble gym

Use these clues to help you unscramble the names of immunomodulatory cytokines used to treat cancer. Then use the circled letters to answer the question posed.

Question: Immunomodulatory cytokines are considered what type of intracellular proteins?

1. Cytokines that primarily interact with leukocytes; one type in particular stimulates the proliferation and cytologic activity of T cells and natural killer cells

S L I N K E U T I N E R

_ _ _ Ⓞ _ _ _ _ _ _ _ Ⓞ

2. Natural substances that stimulate the growth of different types of cells found in the blood and immune system; they have been especially helpful in patients receiving myelosuppressive therapy

L O O N C Y – A M I T T L U N G I S   S C A T O R F

_ _ _ Ⓞ _ _ - _ _ _ _ _ _ _ _ _ _ Ⓞ   _ _ _ _ _ Ⓞ _

3. Agent with antiviral and antitumorigenic effects that slows cell replication and stimulates an immune response; approved to treat chronic myeloid leukemia, hairy cell leukemia, acquired immunodeficiency syndrome-related Kaposi's sarcoma, low-grade malignant lymphoma, multiple myeloma, and renal cell carcinoma

N O N F I R T R E E   H A L P A

_ _ _ Ⓞ _ _ Ⓞ _ _ _   _ _ _ _ _

4. Investigational drug that plays a role in the inflammatory response to tumors and cancer cells; in animal studies, this agent has produced impressive antitumor responses

M U T R O   N O S E S C I R   O C R A F T

_ _ Ⓞ _ _   _ _ _ _ _ _ Ⓞ _ _   _ _ _ _ _ _ _

Answer: __ __ __ __ __ __ __ __ __

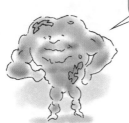

Watch it, tumors—I'm pumped up on immunomodulatory cytokine biological response modifiers! (The drug class name alone should scare 'em, even if my muscles don't.)

▪ Strikeout

These statements pertain to preparation of chemotherapeutic drugs. Cross out the incorrect statement.

1. Many facilities use existing guidelines as the basis for their policies and procedures regarding chemotherapeutic drug preparation and administration.

2. The major sources of chemotherapy guidelines include the American Medical Association, The Centers for Disease Control and Prevention, and the International System of Units.

3. Most health care facilities require nurses and pharmacists who prepare and work with chemotherapeutic drugs to complete a certification program.

4. Preparation of chemotherapeutic drugs requires adherence to guidelines regarding drug preparation areas and equipment, protective clothing, and specific safety measures.

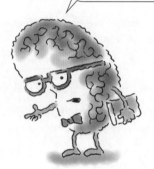

It doesn't take a rocket scientist to know that chemotherapy guidelines exist for the safety of patients and the health care professionals who must prepare and administer such highly toxic drugs.

▪ Mind sprints

In less than 1 minute, list three professionals who may be legally permitted to prepare chemotherapeutic drugs, depending on the state in which they practice.

▪ _____

▪ _____

▪ _____

■ You make the call

Identify these two pieces of equipment and briefly explain why they're needed when working with chemotherapeutic drugs.

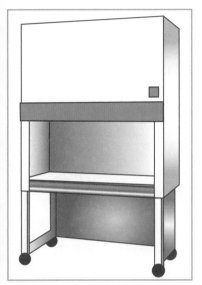

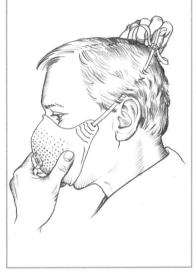

Why they're used: _____

_____

_____

_____

_____

1. _____   2. _____

■ Gear up!

Check off which equipment the Occupational Safety and Health Administration recommends having on hand in the workplace whenever you prepare chemotherapeutic drugs.

☐ 20G needles
☐ 70% alcohol
☐ Alcohol pads
☐ Appropriate diluent (if necessary)
☐ Chemotherapy gloves
☐ Chemotherapy spill kit
☐ Extension tubing
☐ Face shield or goggles and face mask
☐ Hazardous waste container
☐ Hydrophobic filter or dispensing pin
☐ Infusion pump
☐ I.V. containers and tubing
☐ I.V. pole

☐ Long-sleeved gown
☐ Medication labels
☐ Patient's medication order or record
☐ Patient-controlled analgesia pump
☐ Plasma and whole blood
☐ Plastic bags with "hazardous drug" labels
☐ Prescribed drugs
☐ Sharps container
☐ Sterile gauze pads
☐ Syringes with luer-lock fittings
☐ Tourniquet
☐ Venipuncture device

Memory jogger

To remember the clothing you should wear when preparing chemotherapeutic drugs, think of the three G's:

G: _____

G: _____

G: _____

■ Hit or miss

Mark each statement about protective clothing with a "T" for "True" or an "F" for "False."

_____ 1. Gowns should be short-sleeved and made of lint-free cotton that can be easily laundered.

_____ 2. Gloves designed for use with chemotherapeutic drugs should be disposable and made of thick latex or thick non-latex material.

_____ 3. Chemotherapy gloves should be lightly powdered for easy removal, especially when caustic substances are used.

_____ 4. Double gloving should never be done because this makes handling drugs more difficult.

_____ 5. Gloves should be changed whenever a puncture or tear occurs.

_____ 6. Washing your hands before putting on chemotherapy gloves is unnecessary.

_____ 7. You should always put on protective clothing before you begin to compound chemotherapeutic drugs, and always remove your protective gear before leaving the area where the drugs were prepared.

■ Strikeout

These statements pertain to safety measures for working with chemotherapeutic drugs. Cross out all of the incorrect statements.

1. You should use a clean cloth and a mild soap detergent to clean the work surface of the safety cabinet before preparing drugs and after any spills.

2. If a chemotherapeutic drug comes in contact with your skin, you should wash the skin thoroughly with soap and water to prevent absorption into the skin.

3. If a drug comes in contact with your eye, you should immediately flood the eye with isopropyl alcohol while holding the eyelid open.

4. You should report any accident involving chemotherapeutic drugs immediately to your supervisor.

5. You should use blunt-ended needles whenever possible, and use needles with a hydrophobic filter to remove solutions from vials.

6. You should vent vials with a hydrophobic filter or use the negative pressure technique to reduce the amount of aerosolized drugs.

7. If you break an ampule, you should wrap a gauze pad around the neck of the vial to reduce the chance of droplet contamination and glove puncture.

8. You should avoid using syringes and I.V. sets with luer-lock fittings; these can be difficult to remove and may cause a spill.

9. You should always recap needles before putting them in a sharps container.

10. You should transport all prepared chemotherapy drugs in a sealable plastic bag that's prominently labeled with a yellow chemotherapy biohazard label.

■ Boxing match

List some of the items found in a chemotherapy spill kit by writing in answers to these clues, using syllables from the boxes below. The number of syllables for each answer appears in parentheses. Use each syllable only once.

C A N T	C O V	C Y	D E R	D E R	D E S	D U S T
E R S	F R E E	G L E S	G L O V E S	G O G	I C	M A S K
P A N	P I	P O W	P O W	R A	R E S	S H O E
S I	T O	T O R	T O X			

1. Two for your feet (3) __ __ __ __   __ __ __ __ __

2. One for your face (5) __ __ __ __ __ __ __ __ __   __ __ __ __

3. One set to protect your eyes (2) __ __ __ __ __ __ __

4. Two pairs for your hands (4) __ __ __ __ __ __ - __ __ __ __
   __ __ __ __ __

5. A disposable one of these to use with a plastic scraper for collecting broken glass (2) __ __ __ __ __ __ __

6. Used to absorb wet contents; may also use granules instead (5) __ __ __ __ __ __ __ __ __
   __ __ __ __ __

7. Two large waste disposal bags specially designed to safeguard against this type of hazardous material (4) __ __ __ __ __ __ __ __ __

Pep talk

"In creating, the only hard thing is to begin: a grass blade's no easier to make than an oak.

—James Russell Lowell

◼ Starting lineup

Show that you know the proper protocol to follow in the event of a chemotherapy spill by putting these steps in their correct sequence.

Use the disposable dustpan and scraper to collect broken glass or dessicant absorbing powder.	
Carefully place the dustpan, scraper, and collected spill in a leakproof, puncture-proof, chemotherapy-designated hazardous waste container.	
Put on protective garments, if you aren't already wearing them.	
Clean the spill area with a detergent or bleach solution.	
Isolate the area and contain the spill with absorbent materials from the spill kit.	

Pep talk

"As to diseases, make a habit of two things—to help, or at least, to do no harm.
—Hippocrates

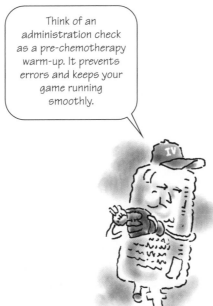

Think of an administration check as a pre-chemotherapy warm-up. It prevents errors and keeps your game running smoothly.

Batter's box

Fill in the missing information on what to do during a preadministration check by using answers from the options box.

Before administering a chemotherapeutic drug, always double-check the order with another

_____ . Also check the patient's _____ before starting the
　　　　1　　　　　　　　　　　　　　　　　　　2

infusion, since many facilities require notifying the practitioner if the count drops below a

predetermined value. Chemotherapeutic drugs that are excreted through the kidneys, such

as cisplatin and carboplatin, also require you to check _____ levels.
　　　　　　　　　　　　　　　　　　　　　　　　　　　　　3

　　It's important to understand which drugs are to be given; whether they're classified as

vesicants, _____ , or irritants; and by which route they should be
　　　　　　　　4

administered.

　　Confirm any written orders for _____ to counteract nausea; additional
　　　　　　　　　　　　　　　　　　　5

fluids; _____ ; or electrolyte supplements to be given before, during, or after
　　　　　6

chemotherapy administration. Verify the patient's level of understanding of the treatment

and _____ . Make sure that either the patient or a legally authorized person
　　　　7

has signed an _____ for each specific chemotherapy drug and for the
　　　　　　　　8

insertion of the I.V. device, if needed.

Options
A. adverse effects
B. antiemetics
C. blood count
D. chemotherapy certified nurse
E. diuretics
F. informed consent form
G. nonvesicants
H. serum creatinine

■ Power stretch

Stretch your knowledge of chemotherapy by first unscrambling the words at left to reveal the three categories in which chemotherapy drugs are grouped based on their risk of tissue damage. Then draw a line from the boxes to their corresponding descriptions and drug examples at right.

SCINTVASE

_ _ _ _ _ _ _ _ _

AVENNOSSTICN

_ _ _ _ _ _ _ _ _ _ _ _

RINSTAIRT

_ _ _ _ _ _ _ _ _

A. Cause a local venous response, with or without a skin reaction

B. Cause a reaction so severe that blisters form and tissue is damaged or destroyed

C. Include asparaginase, bleomycin, cyclophosphamide, cytarabine, floxuridine, and fluorouracil

D. Include carboplatin, carmustine, dacarbazine, etoposide, ifosfamide, irinotecan, streptozocin, and topotecan

E. Cause no irritation or tissue damage

F. Include dactinomycin, daunorubicin, doxorubicin, idarubicin, mechlorethamine, mitomycin, mitoxantrone, nitrogen mustard, vinblastine, vincristine, and vinorelbine

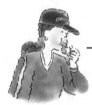

Coaching session
Preventing chemotherapy-related errors

Take these precautions to prevent errors during administration of chemotherapeutic drugs:
• Make sure that orders have been written by only a person qualified to prescribe chemotherapeutic drugs, such as the attending doctor or oncology fellow who's responsible for the patient's care and most familiar with the drug regimen and dosing schedule.
• Double-check all orders before preparing or administering chemotherapeutic drugs.

• Repeatedly check the five "rights" of drug administration: right drug, right patient, right time, right dosage, and right route.
• Question any order that's contrary to customary practice or to the patient's past routine, especially when unusually high dosages or unusual schedules are involved.
• Don't permit any distractions while checking an order or administering treatment.

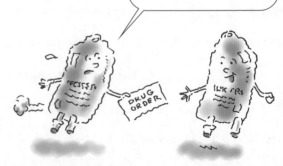

Always take the time to double-check the drug order and the patient's blood count before administering chemotherapeutic drugs.

■■ ■ Hit or miss

Mark each of these statements about infusing chemotherapeutic drugs with a "T" for "True" or an "F" for "False."

_____ 1. Butterfly needles shouldn't be used for infusing chemotherapeutic drugs because they pose an extremely high risk for infiltration.

_____ 2. When gathering equipment, you should make sure you include an extravasation kit if you're administering a nonvesicant or an irritant drug.

_____ 3. You should always select a venous access device with the largest possible gauge when administering chemotherapeutic drugs through a peripheral vein.

_____ 4. Patients receiving continuous vesicant infusions or multiple cycles of chemotherapeutic drugs and patients with poor vein access may require an implanted port.

_____ 5. A high-pressure infusion pump is commonly used to administer vesicant drugs.

_____ 6. I.V. chemotherapeutic drugs can be administered by I.V. push into the infusion device, by indirect I.V. push through the side port of a running I.V. line, or by continuous infusion.

_____ 7. You should always flush the vein with normal saline solution between the administration of each drug during a chemotherapy infusion.

■■ ■ You make the call

Identify the equipment shown in the illustration, and explain why you should have it on hand when administering chemotherapeutic drugs.

Equipment: _____

■ _____
■ _____
■ _____
■ _____
■ _____
■ _____
■ _____
■ _____

Why it's needed: _____

_____

_____

_____

_____

■ Strikeout

Choosing the right vein for chemotherapy can be a tricky process. Cross out all of the incorrect statements below.

1. You should always fully assess the patient's hands and forearms before choosing an appropriate vein.

2. Because chemotherapeutic drugs are so caustic, you should only select a vein that's hard and rigid.

3. You should insert the I.V. catheter proximal to recent puncture sites to prevent the drug from leaking through previously accessed sites.

4. You should avoid upper extremities that have impaired venous circulation.

5. Arms with functioning arteriovenous shunts, grafts, or fistulas for dialysis are obviously strong and therefore good candidates for chemotherapy infusions.

6. To avoid damage to the superficial nerves and tendons, you should use veins in the antecubital fossa and the back of the hand.

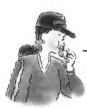

Coaching session
Preventing infiltration

To prevent infiltration when giving vesicants, follow these guidelines:
- Use a distal vein that allows successive proximal venipunctures.
- Avoid using the hand, antecubital space, damaged areas, or areas with compromised circulation.
- Don't probe or "fish" for veins.
- Place a transparent dressing over the site.
- Start the push delivery or the infusion with free-flowing normal saline solution.
- Inspect the site for swelling or erythema.
- Tell the patient to report signs and symptoms of infiltration immediately.
- After administration, flush the line with 20 ml of normal saline solution.

Remember, when it comes to veins, there's no fishing allowed!

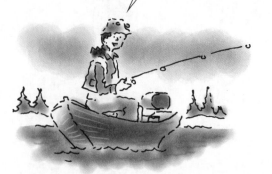

Starting lineup

Show that you know the proper procedure to follow after removing an I.V. line used for chemotherapy by putting these steps in the correct order.

Dispose of unused medications, considered hazardous waste, according to your facility's policy.	
Wash your hands thoroughly with soap and water, even though you have worn gloves.	
Dispose of all needles and contaminated sharps in the red sharps container.	
Put on protective clothing when handling the patient's body fluids for 48 hours after treatment.	
Dispose of personal protective gear, glasses, and gloves in the yellow chemotherapy waste container.	
Document the following: sequence in which drugs were administered; site accessed, gauge and length of catheter, and number of attempts; name, dose, and route of administered drugs; type and volume of I.V. solutions; and any adverse reactions and nursing interventions.	

What makes chemotherapy so effective in killing cancer cells can be equally toxic to normal cells like me. Boy, that stuff really knocks me out!

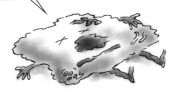

Mind sprints

In 30 seconds, list the three most common infusion-site-related complications of chemotherapy.

- _____
- _____
- _____

■ Jumble gym

Use these clues to help you unscramble signs and symptoms of complications of chemotherapy. Then unscramble the circled letters to answer the question posed.

When you're finished with this exercise, please stop by and help unscramble me!

Question: Many chemotherapeutic drugs cause what short-term side effect due to the destruction of rapidly dividing cells in the hair shaft or root?

1. Results from nerve compression due to swelling associated with infiltration

T O M P E T N C A R M   Y E N D S M O R

_ _ _ _ O _ _ _ _ _ _   _ _ _ _ _ _ _ _

2. May form on skin if extravasation isn't stopped quickly and properly treated

S L E B R I T S

_ O _ _ _ _ _ _

3. May be a consequence of infusion of an irritant that damages the lining of the vein wall

I V E N   B R O S T H S O I M

_ _ _ _   _ _ _ O _ _ _ _ _

4. Can result from an extreme hypersensitivity reaction or anaphylaxis

S L O S   F O   S O U S E N N C O C S I S

_ _ _ _   _ _   O _ _ _ _ _ _ _ _ _ _ _

5. Causes painful mouth ulcers 3 to 7 days after certain chemotherapeutic drugs are given

A O I S I M T T S T

_ _ _ _ O _ O _ _ _

6. Produces anemia, leucopenia, and thrombocytopenia from damage to stem cells in bone marrow

P I N S Y U L E M O P E R S O S

_ _ O _ _ _ _ O _ _ _ _ _ _ _

Answer: _ _ _ _ _ _ _ _

■ Hit or miss

Mark each statement about complications of chemotherapy with a "T" for "True" or an "F" for "False."

_____ 1. Nausea can appear in three patterns (anticipatory, acute, and delayed), and each has its own cause.

_____ 2. Short-term effects of chemotherapy include organ system dysfunction and secondary malignancy.

_____ 3. Pretreatment with lorazepam is usually effective in preventing anticipatory nausea.

_____ 4. A hypersensitivity reaction can occur only with the first dose of the drug.

_____ 5. Initial signs of extravasation can resemble those of hypersensitivity, such as respiratory distress, pruritus, chest pain, dizziness, and agitation.

_____ 6. Patients who lose their hair during chemotherapy may not have the same hair color or texture once their hair growth resumes.

_____ 7. Alopecia is limited to loss of hair on the head.

_____ 8. Stomatitis can lead to electrolyte imbalances and malnutrition if the patient can't swallow adequate food or fluid.

_____ 9. Diarrhea can be brought on when rapidly dividing cells of the intestinal mucosa are killed by chemotherapeutic drugs.

_____ 10. Bleeding gums, increased bruising, petechiae, hypermenorrhea, tarry stools, hematuria, and coffee-ground emesis are all signs of anemia.

■ Batter's box

Complete the following information on the importance of patient teaching with answers from the options box. Use each option only once.

Not only is cancer a frightening and commonly _____ disease, but its
₁

treatment carries serious _____ as well. Help your patient to gain a sense of
₂

control by explaining each procedure you do and by teaching him effective

_____ for dealing with the sometimes overwhelming fear,
₃

_____ , and unwelcome _____ of chemotherapy. Keep in mind
₄   ₅

that a _____ and strong _____ support will enable your
₆   ₇

patient to better endure the disease and its treatments.

Options
A. adverse effects
B. emotional
C. lethal
D. pain
E. positive attitude
F. risks
G. strategies

■ Match point

Match each adverse effect of chemotherapy on the left with its appropriate patient-teaching instruction on the right.

Effect of chemotherapy

1. Anemia _____
2. Diarrhea _____
3. Extravasation _____
4. Hair loss _____
5. Hypersensitivity _____
6. Infiltration _____
7. Leukopenia _____
8. Nausea and vomiting _____
9. Stomatitis _____
10. Thrombocytopenia _____
11. Vein flare _____

Patient-teaching instruction

A. Apply topical steroids or Silvadene cream to the area, as instructed.

B. Report any feeling of swelling, numbness, tingling, or tightness in the arm immediately.

C. Report any burning pain, aching along the vein or up through the arm, or blotchiness immediately.

D. Take antihistamine and corticosteroids, as ordered, before your next scheduled treatment.

E. Take lorazepam, as ordered, at least 1 hour before arriving for treatment.

F. Wear a hat or head covering to protect against sunburn and heat loss; avoid washing your hair excessively or brushing it.

G. Apply ointment to the rectal area if needed because of irritation.

H. Practice good hygiene, take your temperature regularly, eat a low-microbe diet, and avoid crowds, people with colds or respiratory infections, and fresh fruit, fresh flowers, and plants.

I. Take frequent rests, increase your intake of iron-rich foods, and take a multivitamin as prescribed.

J. Report sudden headaches, avoid cuts and bruises, shave with an electric razor, avoid blowing your nose, stay away from irritants that can trigger sneezing, and don't use a rectal thermometer.

K. Practice good oral hygiene, and take prescribed opioid analgesics and topical anesthetics for pain; suck on ice chips to reduce ulcer formation.

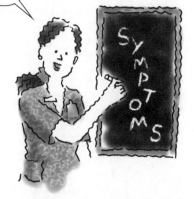

Don't forget to teach your patient the signs and symptoms of all potential adverse effects as well.

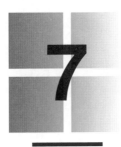

Parenteral nutrition

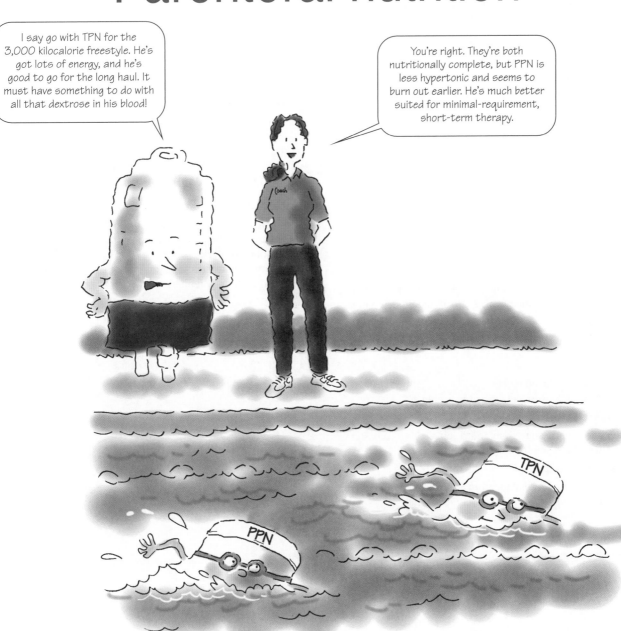

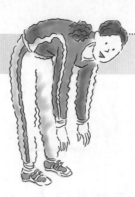

Parenteral nutrition review

Benefits

■ Provides nutrition for patients who can't take nutrients through the GI tract because of illness or surgery
■ Can be used when the patient is hemodynamically unstable or has impaired blood flow to the GI tract

Drawbacks

■ Carries certain risks (catheter infection, hyperglycemia, hypokalemia)
■ Requires vascular access
■ Costs about 10 times more than enteral nutrition

Protein-energy malnutrition

Iatrogenic

■ Inadequate protein and calorie intake during hospitalization

Kwashiorkor

■ Severe protein deficiency without a calorie deficiency
■ Typically occurs in children ages 1 to 3

Marasmus

■ Inadequate intake of protein, calories, and other nutrients
■ Typically occurs in infants ages 6 to 18 months, in patients with mouth and esophageal cancer, and after gastrectomy

Assessing nutritional status

Dietary history

■ Check for decreased intake.
■ Check for increased metabolic requirements.

Physical assessment

■ Check for subtle signs of malnutrition.
■ Obtain anthropometric measurements.

Diagnostic tests

■ Major indicators of malnutrition are changes in the albumin, prealbumin, transferrin, and triglyceride levels.

TPN vs. PPN

TPN

■ Stands for *total parenteral nutrition*
■ Dextrose 20% to 70%
■ Administered through a central line
■ May be given in a 3-L bag with lipids daily
■ Requires starting slow infusion with gradual increase

PPN

■ Stands for *peripheral parenteral nutrition*
■ Dextrose 5% to 10%
■ Administered through a peripheral line
■ Requires larger volume of fluid to meet nutritional needs
■ Doesn't require starting with slow infusion rate

Potential complications

■ Problems related to catheter (clotting, dislodgment, infection, pneumothorax, damaged tubing)
■ Metabolic problems
■ Mechanical complications (air embolism, venous thrombosis, extravasation, phlebitis)

Boxing match

Use syllables in the boxes below to fill in answers to the following clues about parenteral nutrition. The number of syllables for each answer is shown in parentheses. Use each syllable only once.

A C	A L	C A L	C E N	C E S S	G A S	H Y	I	I N	L I S M
K I L	M E	M E N	N A L	N O U S	O	O	O	P E R	R I E S
T A	T A B	T E S	T I	T I O N	T R A L	T R O	V E		

1. Another name for the administration of parenteral solutions (7) _ _ _ _ _ _ _ _ _ _ _ _ _ _ _ _ _ _

2. Units by which energy is measured (5) _ _ _ _ _ _ _ _ _ _ _ _

3. Chemical process by which the body converts food into energy (4) _ _ _ _ _ _ _ _ _

4. Parenteral solutions are needed when the body can't absorb nutrients through this tract (6) _ _ _ _ _ _ _ _ _ _ _ _ _ _ _

5. Method by which long-term high-dextrose parenteral nutrition is delivered (6) _ _ _ _ _ _ _ _ _ _ _ _ _ _ _ _

Parenteral nutrition provides a one-two punch.

It provides the body with basic nutritional support to sustain life, and with the extra energy the body needs to fight infection and disease.

Strikeout

These statements pertain to parenteral nutrition. Cross out all of the incorrect statements.

1. Parenteral nutrition may be used when illness or surgery prevents a patient from eating and metabolizing food.

2. Critically ill patients may receive parenteral nutrition if they're hemodynamically unstable or if the GI tract blood flow is impaired.

3. Essential nutrients in food provide energy, maintain body tissues, and aid body processes such as growth, cell activity, enzyme production, and temperature regulation.

4. A person's caloric requirements depend only on his amount of physical activity.

5. Parenteral solutions can only provide up to one-half of a person's daily nutritional requirements; the rest must come from solid food for metabolism to take place.

6. PPN solutions generally provide more nonprotein calories than TPN solutions.

Cross-training

Complete this crossword puzzle to review some of the terms associated with nutrition and metabolic processes.

Across

3. One of the body's essential proteins needed for metabolism
4. Stands for peripheral delivery of nutrients through a short-term catheter (abbrev.)
7. Having to do with the chemical breakdown of food into energy
8. High blood glucose
9. Low blood potassium; is often a side effect of parenteral nutrition
12. Thirty-foot long tube through which food normally passes in body (two words)
14. Provides total nutritional requirements; given through a central line (abbrev.)
15. Energy units
16. Vein used to access the superior vena cava in central venous infusions

Down

1. Intestinal problem that prevents food contents from passing through the bowel (two words)
2. Another word for *parenteral nutrition*
5. Besides calories, the most common source of nutritional deficiency that can result in malnutrition
6. Biomolecules needed by the body in tiny amounts; are usually provided through a balanced diet but included in parenteral solutions
10. Disease state caused by improper or insufficient diet
11. Glucose solution that provides most of the caloric requirements in parenteral solutions
12. Another term for "fats"

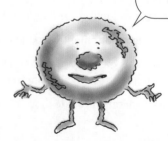

Whether it's dietary or parenteral, a cell's gotta do what a cell's gotta do to get some nutrition!

■ Mind sprints

A parenteral solution may be a specially prepared solution containing at least two nutritional substances. In less than 2 minutes, list the seven key ingredients parenteral solutions commonly contain.

■ _____
■ _____
■ _____
■ _____
■ _____
■ _____
■ _____

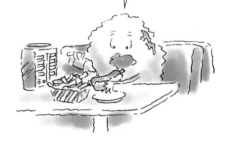

All I have to say about the key ingredients in this culinary delight is 'No comment'!

■ Hit or miss

Mark each of these statements about the advantages and disadvantages of parenteral nutrition with a "T" for "True" or an "F" for "False."

_____ 1. Common conditions that benefit from the use of parenteral nutrition include pancreatitis, ileus, inflammatory bowel disease, GI obstructions, severe malabsorption, and short-bowel syndrome.

_____ 2. Complications of parenteral nutrition include catheter infection, hypoglycemia, and hypokalemia.

_____ 3. Careful monitoring of the catheter site, infusion rate, and laboratory test results can minimize the risks associated with parenteral solutions.

_____ 4. Parenteral nutrition is especially helpful because it allows the cells to function despite the patient's inability to take in or metabolize food through the GI tract.

_____ 5. Central venous access is used for delivering long-term TPN primarily because the solution must be administered at a rapid flow rate.

_____ 6. Parenteral nutrition is beneficial because it's less expensive than enteral feedings.

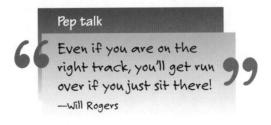

Pep talk

" Even if you are on the right track, you'll get run over if you just sit there! "
—Will Rogers

Power stretch

Stretch your knowledge of parenteral nutrition by first unscrambling the words on the left to reveal two types of commonly administered infusions. Then draw a line from each infusion to its corresponding indications on the right. (Note: each infusion will have more than one indication.)

A. Debilitating illness lasting longer than 2 weeks

B. Poor tolerance of long-term enteral feedings

C. Need of supplemental support without weight gain

D. Deficient or absent oral intake for longer than 7 days (as in multiple trauma, severe burns, or anorexia nervosa)

E. Loss of at least 10% of pre-illness weight

F. Inability to sustain adequate weight with oral or enteral feedings

G. GI disorders that prevent or severely reduce absorption (bowel obstruction, Crohn's disease, ulcerative colitis, short-bowel syndrome, cancer malabsorption syndrome, bowel fistulas)

H. Minimal calorie and protein requirements

I. Supplement to low-calorie intake of oral or enteral feedings

J. Supplement when patient can't absorb enteral feedings

K. Inflammatory bowel disorders (wound infection, fistulas, abscesses)

L. Chronic diarrhea or vomiting

M. Serum albumin level below 3.5 g/dl

```
HARPLIPEER
REALRTENAP
TONUTINRI

__ __ __ __ __ __ __ __ __ __
__ __ __ __ __ __ __ __ __ __
__ __ __ __ __ __ __ __ __
```

```
ATTLO   TERRAPLANE
RUNTOITNI

__ __ __ __ __ __
__ __ __ __ __ __ __ __ __ __
__ __ __ __ __ __ __ __ __
```

Here's the skinny on parenteral nutrition. You should use it cautiously in patients with severe liver damage, coagulation disorders, anemia, and pulmonary disease and those at increased risk for fat embolism.

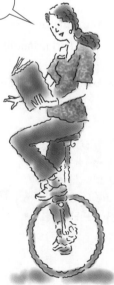

Pep talk

" Champions aren't made in gyms. Champions are made from something they have deep inside them: A desire, a dream, a vision. They have to have last-minute stamina, they have to be a little faster, they have to have the skill and the will. But the will must be stronger than the skill. "

—Muhammad Ali

■■
■ Batter's box

Fill in the missing information about nutritional deficiencies with answers from these options.

The most common nutritional deficiencies involve _____ and calories.

1

Nutritional deficiencies may result from a _____ GI tract, decreased food

2

intake, increased _____ need, or a combination of these factors. Food intake

3

may be decreased because of _____ , decreased _____ , or

4   5

injury. Decreased food intake may also occur with GI disorders, such as

_____ , surgery, or sepsis.

6

An increase in metabolic activity requires increased _____ . A

7

_____ commonly increases metabolic activity. The metabolic rate may also

8

increase in victims of _____ , trauma, disease, or stress; patients may

9

require twice the calories of their _____ (the minimum energy needed to

10

maintain _____ , circulation, and other basic body functions).

11

Options
A. basal metabolic rate
B. burns
C. caloric intake
D. fever
E. illness
F. metabolic
G. nonfunctional
H. paralytic ileus
I. physical ability
J. protein
K. respiration

As a last resort, the body fights starvation by breaking down my reserves in bone, muscle, and other tissues. Parenteral nutrition can prevent this.

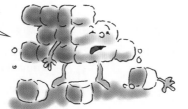

■■
■ Circuit training

When the body detects protein-calorie deficiency, it turns to its reserve sources of energy. Draw arrows between the squares below to show the order in which the body draws upon these energy reserves.

The body draws energy from the fats stored in adipose tissue.

The body taps its store of essential visceral proteins (serum albumin and transferrin) and somatic body proteins (skeletal, smooth muscle, and tissue proteins). These proteins and their amino acids are converted to glucose for energy through a process called *gluconeogenesis*.

The body mobilizes and converts glycogen to glucose through a process called *glycogenolysis*.

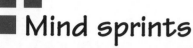

Mind sprints

List five disorders that can lead to protein-energy malnutrition as a result of inadequate calorie intake or high metabolic protein and energy requirements. See if you can list all five in 1 minute or less.

- _____
- _____
- _____
- _____
- _____

Power stretch

Stretch your knowledge of protein-energy malnutrition (PEM) by first unscrambling the words on the left to reveal three types of PEM. Then draw a line from each type to its characteristics on the right.

A. Results from severe protein deficiency without a calorie deficit

B. Occurs because of inadequate protein or calorie intake, commonly during hospitalization

C. Usually is secondary to malabsorption disorders, cancer and cancer therapies, kidney disease, hypermetabolic illness, or iatrogenic causes

D. Characterized by a prolonged, gradual wasting of muscle mass and subcutaneous fat

E. Affects more than 15% of patients in acute care settings

F. Most commonly affects children ages 1 to 3

G. Caused by an inadequate intake of protein, calories, and other nutrients

H. Occurs most commonly in infants ages 6 to 18 months, after gastrectomy, and in patients with cancer of the mouth and esophagus

I. Occurs most commonly in patients hospitalized more than 2 weeks

SMARUMSA

— — — — — — — —

GRITIOCEAN

— — — — — — — — — —

ASKOHIRWORK

— — — — — — — — — — —

■ ■
■ Strikeout

These statements pertain to the nutritional assessment. Cross out the incorrect statements.

1. You can obtain all the information you need for a thorough nutritional assessment based on the information in a patient's dietary history.

2. When obtaining a dietary history, you should check for signs of decreased food intake or increased metabolic requirements (or a combination of the two) and any factors that affect food intake, including appetite.

3. A complete assessment should cover the patient's chief complaint, present illness, medical history, allergies, family history, and lifestyle.

4. The most commonly used anthropometric measurements include the patient's food preferences, personal habits, cultural influences, and religious beliefs.

5. Triceps skinfold thickness, midarm circumference, and midarm muscle circumference are less commonly used anthropometric measurements because they tend to vary by age and race.

6. A finding of less than 90% of the standard anthropometric measurement may indicate a need for nutritional support.

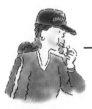

Coaching session
Subtle signs of poor nutrition

During your physical assessment, look for these subtle signs of poor nutrition:
- poor skin turgor
- bruising
- abnormal pigmentation
- darkening of the mouth lining
- protruding eyes (exophthalmos)
- neck swelling
- adventitious breath sounds
- dental caries
- ill-fitting dentures
- signs of infection or irritation in and around the mouth
- muscle wasting
- abdominal wasting, masses, and tenderness
- enlarged liver.

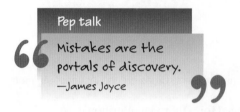

Match point

Laboratory studies help pinpoint nutritional deficiencies by aiding in the diagnosis of anemia, malnutrition, and other disorders. Match the test on the left with its normal adult values on the right.

Test

1. Serum albumin _____
2. Creatinine height index _____
3. Hematocrit _____
4. Hemoglobin _____
5. Serum transferrin _____
6. Serum triglycerides _____
7. Total lymphocyte count _____
8. Total protein screen _____
9. Urine ketone bodies _____
10. Transthyretin (prealbumin) _____

Normal adult values

A. Male: 42% to 50%; female: 40% to 48%

B. 200 to 400 µg/dl

C. 16 to 40 mg/dl

D. 1,500 to 3,000 µl

E. Based on patient's height or weight

F. Male: 13 to 18 g/dl; female: 12 to 16 g/dl

G. 3.5 to 5 g/dl

H. 40 to 200 mg/dl

I. 6 to 8 g/dl

J. Negative for ketones in urine

I'm sure you're aware of it, but I'll remind you anyway. Outside of the commonly ordered laboratory studies, albumin, prealbumin, transferrin, and triglyceride levels are the major indicators of nutritional deficiency.

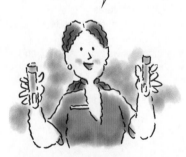

Jumble gym

Use the clues to help you unscramble words related to parenteral nutrition solutions. Then use the circled letters to answer the question posed.

Question: The practitioner may prescribe what other additive to the parenteral nutrition solution when necessary to counteract the effects of infusions with hyperosmolar glucose concentrations?

1. Basic building blocks of protein; used in parenteral solutions to maintain protein stores and to prevent protein loss from muscles

N A I M O   S C I A D

— — —◯— — —◯— —

2. Added to parenteral nutrition solutions based on an evaluation of the patient's serum chemistry profile and metabolic needs

Y E L L O E R S T C T E   D A N   N A I L S R E M

— — — — — —◯— — — — — — — — —◯— — — — — —

3. Also called *trace elements*; added to parenteral solutions to promote normal metabolism; include zinc, copper, chromium, selenium, and manganese

S T I R U C M I T E N N O R

— — — — — —◯— — — —◯— —

4. Provides most of the calories that can help maintain nitrogen balance; exact number of nonprotein calories depends on the severity of the patient's illness

T O X E R D E S

— — — — — —◯—

> Glucose balance is extremely important in a patient receiving TPN. Because I need a little time to adjust to the increased insulin production demands, start infusions slowly and increase them gradually, as ordered.

Answer: __ __ __ __ __ __ __

Mind sprints

We've identified eight factors that can further throw off the glucose balance in a patient receiving a TPN solution. Time yourself and see if you can name them all in 2 minutes or less.

- _____
- _____
- _____
- _____
- _____
- _____
- _____
- _____

■■
■ Hit or miss

Mark each of these statements about TPN with a "T" for "True" or an "F" for "False."

_____ 1. TPN requires surgical implantation of a central venous access device, which can be done at the patient's bedside.

_____ 2. TPN solutions can deliver a large quantity of nutrients and calories (2,000 to 3,000 calories/day or more).

_____ 3. Daily allotments of TPN solutions are commonly given in a single 3-L bag, called a *total nutrient admixture* or a *3:1 solution*.

_____ 4. All TPN infusions should be stopped slowly because abruptly stopping the infusion can cause hyperglycemia.

_____ 5. TPN solutions are hypotonic.

_____ 6. TPN solutions are extremely effective in severely stressed patients, such as those with sepsis or burns.

_____ 7. TPN solutions may interfere with immune mechanisms.

_____ 8. Lipids may be given as a separate solution or as an admixture with dextrose and amino acids in a TPN solution.

> Every additive in a parenteral solution has a specific purpose in helping to maintain metabolism or correct metabolic deficiencies.

■■
■ Match point

Common parenteral solutions contain dextrose 50% in water, amino acids, and various other additives. Match each additive on the left with its purpose on the right.

Additive

1. Acetate _____
2. Calcium _____
3. Chloride _____
4. Folic acid _____
5. Magnesium _____
6. Phosphate _____
7. Potassium _____
8. Sodium _____
9. Vitamin B complex _____
10. Vitamin C _____
11. Vitamin D _____
12. Vitamin K _____

Purpose

A. Aids in the final absorption of carbohydrates and protein

B. Needed for deoxyribonucleic acid formation and to promote growth and development

C. Minimizes the potential for developing peripheral paresthesia (numbness and tingling of extremities)

D. Prevents metabolic acidosis

E. Promotes development of bones and teeth and aids blood clotting

F. Prevents bleeding disorders

G. Regulates the acid-base equilibrium and maintains osmotic pressure

H. Helps in wound healing

I. Is essential for bone metabolism and maintenance of serum calcium levels

J. Aids carbohydrate and protein absorption

K. Helps regulate water distribution and maintain normal fluid balance

L. Needed for cellular activity and tissue synthesis

■■ ■ Mind sprints

Abruptly stopping a patient's parenteral infusion is one way to throw off his glucose balance. In less than 3 minutes, list the other factors that can change a patient's glucose balance.

- _____
- _____
- _____
- _____
- _____
- _____
- _____
- _____

> Like TPN, PPN solutions are nutritionally complete but usually lower in calories and given only short-term.

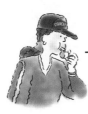

■■ ■ Strikeout

This information pertains to PPN solutions. Cross out all of the incorrect statements.

1. PPN solutions are typically given to patients who can tolerate high volumes of fluid, to patients who are expected to resume bowel function and oral feedings in a few days, and to those who aren't candidates for central venous access devices.

2. Some PPN solutions are hypertonic, having an osmolarity no higher than 600 mOsm/L.

3. Lipid emulsions, electrolytes, trace elements, and vitamins may be added to a PPN solution to add calories and other needed nutrients.

4. PPN solutions are usually more concentrated than TPN solutions and therefore require less fluid.

5. PPN is best reserved for patients with severe malnutrition or problems with fat metabolism.

6. Lipid emulsions with a concentration of 10% to 20% are nearly isotonic; therefore, they can be safely infused through a peripheral vein as part of PPN.

7. Caring for a patient receiving a PPN infusion involves the same steps required for any patient receiving a peripheral I.V. infusion.

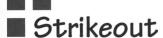

Coaching session
Pros and cons of using 3:1 solutions

A 3:1 solution, or *total nutrient admixture*, is a white solution that delivers a day's worth of nutrients in a single 3-L bag by combining lipids with other parenteral solution components.

The pros
- Requires less bag handling (lowers risk of contamination)
- Requires less time to administer
- Decreases the need for infusion sets and electronic infusion devices
- Lowers hospital costs
- Increases patient mobility
- Eases adjustment to home care

The cons
- Precludes use of certain infusion devices because of their inability to accurately deliver large volumes of solution
- Requires a 1.2-micron filter (rather than a 0.22-micron filter) to allow lipid molecules through
- Limits amount of calcium and phosphorus added because of the difficulty in detecting precipitates in the milky white solution

Power stretch

Stretch your knowledge of parenteral nutrition by first unscrambling the words at left to reveal two ways in which parenteral nutrition solutions are delivered. Then draw a line from each term to its corresponding characteristics on the right. (Note: each term with have more than one characteristic.)

SNOUTICONU
VIDELYRE

— — — — — — — — — — —
— — — — — — — —

CLCYCI
PEARTHY

— — — — — — —
— — — — — — —

A. Given over a period of 8 to 16 hours

B. Begins at a slow rate, then increases to optimal rate as ordered

C. Given over a 24-hour period

D. Commonly used in home care therapy

E. May be used to wean patient from TPN

F. May prevent complications, such as hyperglycemia, caused by a high dextrose load

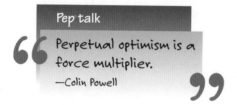

Pep talk

"Perpetual optimism is a force multiplier."
—Colin Powell

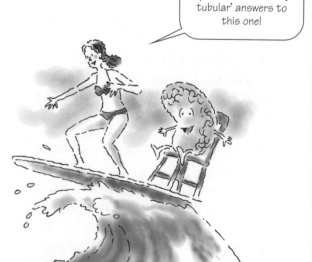

I bet you'll come up with a few 'totally tubular' answers to this one!

Gear up!

Check off which equipment you'll need to gather to administer a TPN solution.

☐ Alcohol swabs
☐ Blood collection kit
☐ Clean gloves
☐ Goggles
☐ Heparin solution
☐ Infusion pump
☐ I.V. administration set (with filtered tubing)
☐ I.V. pole

☐ Mask
☐ Practitioner order
☐ Prescribed TPN solution
☐ Sterile dressings, tape
☐ Stethoscope
☐ Syringe
☐ Thermometer
☐ Venipuncture device
☐ Warming blanket

▪ Hit or miss

Mark each of these statements about administering TPN with a "T" for "True" or an "F" for "False."

_____ 1. Because TPN fluid has about six times the solute concentration of blood, peripheral I.V. administration can cause sclerosis and thrombosis; therefore, central venous access is necessary.

_____ 2. Long-term TPN therapy requires the use of only an implanted port.

_____ 3. Before TPN administration begins, the doctor must insert the access device and confirm by X-ray that the catheter tip is in the superior vena cava.

_____ 4. When setting up equipment, use of a filtered tubing is desired, but optional.

_____ 5. You should administer only chilled TPN solution to ensure freshness and prevent spoiling.

_____ 6. You should always check the written order against the label on the TPN bag or bottle to make sure that the specific volumes, concentrations, and additives are included. Also double-check the infusion rate.

_____ 7. You should always inspect the TPN solution carefully before administering an infusion, and you should notify the pharmacist and the practitioner if you detect anything suspicious.

_____ 8. You should never let a TPN solution hang for longer than 8 hours.

_____ 9. You should adjust the flow rate as needed throughout TPN therapy.

_____ 10. Adding prescribed medications to the TPN container is standard practice in most facilities.

▪ Match point

When administering TPN solutions, always observe the patient for signs and symptoms or infusion-related problems. Match the signs and symptoms on the left with the likely problem on the right.

Signs and symptoms

1. Discomfort (at the start of the infusion) _____

2. Fever, chills, discomfort on infusion, redness or drainage at catheter insertion site _____

3. Fever, pressure sensation over the eyes, nausea, vomiting, headache, chest and back pain, tachycardia, dyspnea, cyanosis, flushing, sweating, chills _____

4. Swelling at catheter insertion site _____

Likely problem

A. Catheter infection

B. Adverse reaction to TPN solution, particularly the lipid emulsion

C. Extravasation of TPN solution

D. Catheter malpositioning or impairment

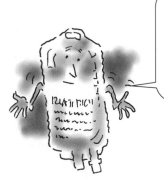

Why take chances? If you detect any clouding, floating debris, or color change in the TPN infusate, report it immediately. It could be contaminated, or there may be a problem with the solution's integrity or pH level.

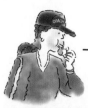

Coaching session
Administering lipid emulsions

Most TPN solutions contain lipid emulsions. Follow these precautions for safe administration:
• Check the solution for separation or an oily appearance. If either condition exists, the lipid may have come out of the emulsion and shouldn't be used.
• Begin with a test dose, monitoring the patient's vital signs and observing for adverse reactions (fever, pressure sensation over eyes, nau-sea and vomiting, headache, chest and back pain, tachycardia, respiratory distress, cyanosis, flushing, sweating, or chills).
• If the patient tolerates the test dose well, begin the infusion at the prescribed rate.
• Discard any leftover solution. Never rehang a partially empty bottle of emulsion because lipid emulsions have a high risk of bacterial growth.

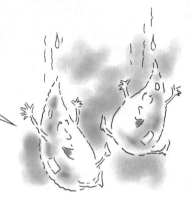

A drop here, a drop there! We tend to accumulate quickly, so make sure you measure accurately.

■ Power stretch

Stretch your knowledge of parenteral nutrition by first unscrambling the words on the left to reveal five nursing assessments required to maintain TPN infusions. Then draw a line from each assessment to its corresponding nursing interventions on the right. (Note: each assessment may have more than one corresponding intervention.)

LIVAT SNIGS

_ _ _ _ _   _ _ _ _ _

EGRIFTSNICK SETT

_ _ _ _ _ _ _ _ _ _ _
_ _ _ _

KITEAN NDA UTOPUT

_ _ _ _ _   _ _ _
_ _ _ _ _ _

BYATROLAOR SETTS

_ _ _ _ _ _ _ _ _ _ _
_ _ _ _ _

A. Record these at the start of therapy and every 4 to 8 hours thereafter (or more frequently if necessary).

B. Monitor results, especially serum electrolyte, blood urea nitrogen, and glucose levels.

C. Be alert for increased body temperature—an early sign of catheter-related sepsis.

D. Keep accurate daily records, specifying volume and type.

E. Perform test as ordered to monitor glucose levels.

F. Check protein and enzyme levels, including cholesterol, triglyceride, and plasma-free fatty acids, weekly.

G. Check for abnormal electrolyte levels indicative of nutritional problems.

H. Use this as a diagnostic tool to assure prompt, precise replacement of fluid and electrolyte deficits.

▪▪ ▪ Strikeout

These statements are patient-teaching instructions you might need to give a patient who will be receiving home TPN therapy. Cross out any instruction that provides incorrect or inaccurate information.

1. "Look for signs of catheter infection during the infusion, such as fever, chills, discomfort, and redness or drainage at the catheter site."

2. "I'll show you how to adjust the flow rate of the I.V. to get it to the rate ordered by the practitioner; once you get it to that rate, you shouldn't need to adjust it further."

3. "A gradual increase in flow rate is necessary to allow the pancreas to adjust to the increased glucose production needed because of the high level of insulin in the treatment."

4. "Throughout your treatment, you'll need to look for signs and symptoms of fluid, electrolyte, and glucose imbalances."

5. "There are very tiny amounts of vitamins and minerals in TPN, so it isn't necessary to look for signs of deficiencies or toxicities."

6. "TPN isn't really a medication, so you don't need to be concerned with incompatibility problems with other drugs."

7. "You should never mix in any other liquids or medications with your TPN solution."

8. "You should always inspect the TPN solution for color changes, floating debris, and cloudiness. Don't use any solution with these problems because it could be contaminated."

▪▪ ▪ Mind sprints

In 1 minute or less, list four things you need to write on the label of a patient's TPN container.

▪ _____
▪ _____
▪ _____
▪ _____

Here's a handy tip: If the TPN bag or bottle is damaged and you don't have an immediate replacement, you can approximate the glucose concentration until a new container is ready by adding 50% glucose to $D_{10}W$.

Pep talk

"Leadership should be born out of the understanding of the needs of those who would be affected by it.

—Marian Anderson

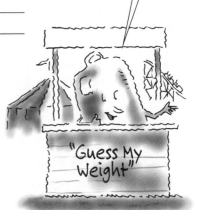

"Guess My Weight"

■ Cross-training

Work out the clues below to complete this crossword puzzle on PPN.

Across

1. Painful inflammation along the vein pathway; often a complication of PPN therapy

5. Method of delivering lipid emulsion when it isn't part of the PPN solution

12. Central vein not used in PPN (three words)

14. Usual length of therapy with PPN (two words)

15. Pancreatic enzyme that increases insulin requirements in those receiving PPN

16. Feeling of fullness often reported by patients receiving PPN

Down

2. These prevent and treat essential fatty acid deficiency and provide a major source of energy (two words).

3. Needed to access vein for PPN infusion

4. Tendency for excessive blood coagulation that may occur with receiving lipid emulsions

6. Swelling at the insertion site may signal this; can lead to tissue damage

7. High lipid levels in the blood

8. Abnormally low platelet count; may occur in patients receiving lipid emulsions

9. Large vein that may be accessed in PPN

10. Because this is lower in PPN solutions than in TPN solutions, the patient must be able to tolerate large volumes of fluid.

11. PPN provides approximately 1,300 to 1,800 of these per day.

13. Found in concentrations of 5% to 10% in PPN

> If you're giving a lipid emulsion separate from the PPN solution, piggyback the lipid emulsion below the in-line filter close to the insertion site. That way, the lipids won't clog the filtration line. Isn't that right?

> You know it!

■ Starting lineup

Show that you know how to switch a patient from continuous to cyclic TPN by putting these steps in their correct order.

Draw a blood glucose sample 1 hour after the infusion ends.	
Reduce the flow rate by one-half for 1 hour before stopping the infusion.	
Observe for signs of hypoglycemia.	
Stop the infusion.	
Begin administering the continuous infusion.	

> When switching from continuous to cyclic TPN, adjust the flow rate so that the patient's blood glucose level can adapt to the decreased nutrient load.

■ Strikeout

These statements pertain to administering lipids and lipid emulsions.
Cross out any incorrect statements.

1. Early adverse reactions to lipid emulsion therapy include fever, difficulty breathing, cyanosis, nausea, vomiting, headache, flushing, sweating, lethargy, dizziness, chest and back pain, slight pressure over the eyes, and irritation at the infusion site.

2. Adverse reactions occur in about one-half of all patients receiving lipid emulsion therapy.

3. Late adverse reactions to lipid therapy include glucose in the urine, chills, malaise, leukocytosis, altered level of consciousness, elevated blood glucose levels, and fever.

4. Because the synthesis of lipase (a fat-splitting enzyme) increases insulin requirements, the insulin dosage of a diabetic patient may need to be increased as ordered.

5. You may need to administer thyroid-stimulating hormone (TSH) to a patient with hypothyroidism who's receiving long-term TPN therapy because TSH affects lipase activity and may prevent triglycerides from accumulating in the vascular system.

6. Lipids are extremely small and easily pass through I.V. tubing when administered as part of parenteral therapy.

7. Many patients receiving lipid emulsions report a feeling of fullness or bloating; occasionally, they experience an unpleasant metallic or greasy taste.

8. Lipid emulsions may clear from the blood at an accelerated rate in someone with severe burns, multiple trauma, or a metabolic imbalance.

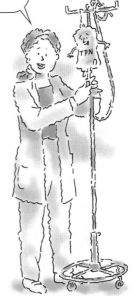

Mind sprints

Children have a greater need than adults for seven nutrients. As fast as you can, name at least five of these nutrients in the spaces provided.

- _____
- _____
- _____
- _____
- _____
- _____
- _____

> **Pep talk**
>
> 66 The known is finite, the unknown infinite; intellectually we stand on an islet in the midst of in illimitable ocean of inexplicability. Our business in every generation is to reclaim a little more land. 99
> —T.H. Huxley

Strikeout

These statements refer to pediatric patients receiving parenteral nutrition. Cross out all of the incorrect statements.

1. Parenteral feeding therapy for children serves a dual purpose: maintaining the child's nutritional status while preventing inborn errors of metabolism.

2. Health care providers should keep these factors in mind when planning to meet a child's nutritional needs: age, weight, activity level, size, development, and calorie needs.

3. Administering TPN with lipid emulsions in a premature or low-birth-weight neonate may lead to lipid accumulation in the lungs.

4. Hypoproteinemia can occur in infants receiving 20% lipid emulsions.

I may not look like one, but in some circles I'm considered a superhero—especially among pediatric and elderly patients, who are particularly susceptible to fluid overload and heart failure.

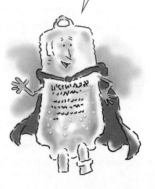

Power stretch

Stretch your knowledge of complications of TPN by first unscrambling the words on the left to reveal five common catheter-related problems. Then draw a line from each problem to its corresponding interventions on the right. (Note: each problem may have more than one intervention.)

SPESSI

— — — — — —

DOLTECT HETTRACE

— — — — — — —
— — — — — — — — —

REACTETH DEEDGLINTMOS

— — — — — — —
— — — — — — — — — —

CRECKAD BITGUN

— — — — — — —
— — — — — —

REXMUPHOTNOA

— — — — — — — — — — —

A. Apply a padded hemostat above the break to prevent air from entering the line.

B. Assist with chest tube insertion.

C. Instill alteplase (t-PA) to clear the catheter lumen as ordered.

D. Remove the catheter, and culture the tip.

E. Give appropriate antibiotics.

F. Reposition the catheter.

G. Place a sterile gauze pad treated with antimicrobial ointment on the insertion site, and apply pressure.

H. Maintain chest tube suctioning as ordered.

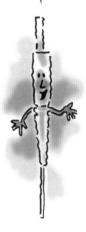

Always look for obvious indications of a problem as well as physiologic signs that something may be wrong.

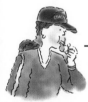

Coaching session
Spotting catheter-related problems

Sometimes it's easy to spot catheter-related problems, such as when a catheter becomes dislodged from a vein. In some cases, you'll need to look for more subtle signs of a problem.

Catheter dislodgment
• Wet dressing
• Patient's report of feeling cold or that gown is wet
• Redness or swelling around the insertion site (can occur from extravasation of solution in both PPN and TPN)

• Bleeding from the insertion site
• Signs and symptoms of air embolism (respiratory distress, unequal breath sounds, weak pulse, increased central venous pressure, decreased blood pressure, loss of consciousness)

Damaged catheter, access device, or tubing
• Infusate leaking from the cracked area or insertion site (can occur with damaged catheter or access device)
• Infusate leaking from damaged area

while insertion site remains dry (damaged tubing)

Pneumothorax
• Dyspnea, chest pain, cough, cyanosis
• Diminished breath sounds
• Sweating
• Unilateral chest movement

Sepsis
• Unexplained fever, chills, and a red, indurated area around catheter site
• Unexplained hyperglycemia

Match point

Metabolic complications of parenteral nutrition result from physiological causes brought on by the infusion. Match the complication on the left with likely cause on the right.

Complication

1. Hyperglycemia _____
2. Hypocalcemia _____
3. Hypoglycemia _____
4. Liver dysfunction _____
5. Hypomagnesemia _____
6. Hyperkalemia _____
7. Hyperosmolar hyperglycemic nonketotic syndrome (HHNS) _____
8. Hypokalemia _____
9. Hypophosphatemia _____
10. Metabolic acidosis _____

Likely cause

A. Caused by hyperosmolar diuresis from untreated hyperglycemia

B. Results from too little potassium in the solution, excessive loss of potassium brought on by GI tract disturbances or diuretic use, or large doses of insulin

C. Caused by too little magnesium in the solution

D. Can develop if the formula's glucose concentration is excessive, the infusion rate is too rapid, or glucose tolerance is compromised by diabetes, stress, or sepsis

E. Results when therapy is suddenly disrupted or the patient receives excessive insulin

F. Caused by too much potassium in the formula, renal disease, or hyponatremia

G. Develops from an increased serum chloride level and a decreased bicarbonate level

H. Results from insulin therapy and inadequate phosphate in the solution; also associated with conditions such as alcoholism that can lead to malnutrition

I. Results from long-term use of solution that tends to raise serum alkaline phosphatase, lactate dehydrogenase, and bilirubin levels

J. Caused by too little calcium in the solution, vitamin D deficiency, or pancreatitis

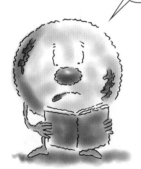

Wow! The list of complications is nearly as long as the list of ingredients on the TPN container!

> ## Pep talk
>
> To be nobody but yourself in a world which is doing its best day and night to make you everybody else means to fight the hardest battle which any human being can fight, and never stop fighting.
>
> —e.e. cummings

Team up!

Always be on the lookout for signs and symptoms of hyperglycemia and hypoglycemia in a patient receiving parenteral nutrition. Put each of these signs and symptoms under the correct heading. Use all of the terms in the box; one term will appear under both columns.

Hyperglycemia (high blood glucose)

_____

_____

_____

_____

_____

_____

Hypoglycemia (low blood glucose)

_____

_____

_____

_____

Signs and symptoms
- Anxiety
- Coma
- Confusion
- Deliriousness
- Fatigue
- Irritability
- Restlessness
- Shaking
- Sweating
- Weakness

I'll just hang out here while you solve this one!

Match point

Test you assessment skills by matching the complications of parenteral nutrition on the left with the corresponding signs and symptoms on the right.

Complications

1. HHNS _____

2. Hyperkalemia _____

3. Hypokalemia _____

4. Hypomagnesemia _____

5. Hypophosphatemia _____

6. Hypocalcemia _____

Signs and symptoms

A. Muscle weakness, paralysis, paresthesia, cardiac arrhythmias

B. Numbing or tingling sensations, tetany, polyuria, dehydration, arrhythmias

C. Skeletal muscle weakness, decreased heart rate, irregular pulse, tall T waves

D. Glycosuria, electrolyte disturbances, confusion, lethargy, seizures, possibly coma

E. Tingling around mouth, paresthesia in fingers, mental changes, hyperreflexia, tetany, arrhythmias

F. Irritability, weakness, paresthesia; in extreme cases, coma and cardiac arrest

■ Answers

■ Chapter 1

■ Page 4

Batter's box

1. E, C, or H, 2. E, C, or H, 3. E, C, or H, 4. G, 5. B, 6. F, 7. A,
8. I, 9. D

■ Page 5

Boxing match

2. Overdose, 3. Incompatibility, 4. Infection, 5. Bleeding

Hit or miss

1. False. It's roughly 60% of total body weight.
2. True.
3. True.
4. False. The major compartments are ICF and ECF.
5. False. Fluid distribution normally remains constant between the compartments.
6. True.
7. False. Intravascular fluid accounts for most of the blood volume.
8. True.
9. False. It occurs with a 2% loss.
10. True.

■ Page 6

Mind sprints

Fluid deficit
- Weight loss
- Increased, thready pulse rate
- Diminished blood pressure
- Decreased central venous pressure
- Sunken eyes, dry conjunctivae, decreased tearing
- Poor skin turgor
- Pale, cool skin
- Poor capillary refill
- Lack of moisture in groin and axillae
- Thirst
- Dry mouth, dry, cracked lips
- Furrows in tongue
- Difficulty forming words
- Mental status changes
- Weakness
- Diminished urine output
- Increased hematocrit, serum electrolyte levels
- Blood urea nitrogen levels
- Serum osmolarity

Fluid excess
- Weight gain
- Elevated blood pressure
- Bounding pulse
- Jugular vein distention
- Increased respiratory rate
- Dyspnea
- Moist crackles or rhonchi
- Edema
- Puffy eyelids
- Periorbital edema
- Slow emptying of hand veins when arm is raised
- Decreased hematocrit, blood urea nitrogen levels, and serum osmolarity

Strikeout

2. ~~Electrolyte imbalances rarely cause problems because the body can tolerate wide extremes in electrolyte levels.~~ The body's homeostasis is dependent on keeping electrolyte levels in close control, and it can't tolerate wide extremes in these levels.
5. ~~Electrolytes are measured only in units of milliequivalents per liter (mEq/L).~~ Electrolytes are also measured in milligrams per deciliter (mg/dl).
6. ~~A cation is an electrolyte with a negative charge.~~ An electrolyte with a negative charge is an anion.

■ Page 7

Match point

1. D, 2. F, 3. A, 4. B, 5. E, 6. C

■ Page 8

Power stretch

Hypocalcemia: B Hypernatremia: C
Hyperkalemia: D Hypokalemia: E
Hyponatremia: A

Memory jogger

Hypo-: low, below normal

Hyper-: high, above normal

Iso-: equal, uniform

■ Page 9

Batter's box

1. D, 2. B, 3. C, 4. A or E, 5. A or E, 6. F

■ Page 10

Power stretch

Osmosis: C, D, F, J

Diffusion: A, C, D

Active transport: B, H, I

Capillary diffusion: E, G, I, K

You make the call

Process: Capillary filtration

What's happening: Hydrostatic pressure builds and forces fluids and solutes through a semipermeable membrane.

■ Page 11

Cross-training

■ Page 12

Hit or miss

1. True.
2. True.
3. False. Osmolarity is about 300 mOsm/L.
4. False. It suggests fluid overload, such as hypervolemia.
5. True.

Match point

1. C, 2. B, 3. A

■ Page 13

You make the call

1. Type of solution: **Hypotonic solution**

   How it changes/maintains body fluid status: Shifts fluid out of the intravascular compartment, hydrating the cell and the interstitial compartments

2. Type of solution: **Isotonic solution**

   How it changes/maintains body fluid status: Stays in the intravascular space, expanding the intravascular compartment without pulling fluid from other compartments

3. Type of solution: **Hypertonic solution**

   How it changes/maintains body fluid status: Draws fluid into the intravascular compartment from the cells and the interstitial compartments

■ Page 14

Team up!

Isotonic
- 5% albumin
- dextrose 5% in water
- Hetastarch
- lactated Ringer's
- normal saline
- Normosol
- Ringer's

Hypotonic
- dextrose 2.5% in water
- half-normal saline
- 0.33% sodium chloride

Hypertonic
- 25% albumin
- dextrose 5% in half-normal saline
- dextrose 5% in lactated Ringer's
- dextrose 5% in normal saline
- 3% sodium chloride
- 7.5% sodium chloride

Strikeout

3. ~~Reduce fluid in the circulation~~
5. ~~Hydrate the cells~~
6. ~~Increase intracranial pressure (ICP)~~

■ Page 15

Batter's box

1. G, 2. A, 3. B, 4. I, 5. D, 6. E, 7. F, 8. C, 9. J, 10. H

■ **Page 16**
Jumble gym

1. Cardiovascular drugs
2. Antibiotics
3. Thrombolytics
4. Histamine-receptor antagonists
5. Antineoplastics
6. Anticonvulsants

Answer: Intermittent

■ **Page 17**
Mind sprints

- Proteins
- Carbohydrates
- Fats
- Electrolytes
- Vitamins
- Trace elements
- Water

Strikeout

2. ~~A patient can receive TPN only up to 6 months.~~ A patient can receive TPN indefinitely.
4. ~~Peripheral parenteral nutrition (PPN) can be given indefinitely.~~ PPN can only be given for approximately 3 weeks because of the risk to the veins.
8. ~~Because TPN doesn't contain sugar, it isn't necessary to check the patient's glucose levels.~~ TPN contains high levels of glucose, so you should keep close track of changes in his fluid and electrolyte status and glucose levels.

■ **Page 18**
Batter's box

1. C, 2. E, 3. D, 4. A, 5. B

Train your brain

Answer: Continuous I.V. infusion helps maintain a constant therapeutic drug level.

■ **Page 19**
Finish line

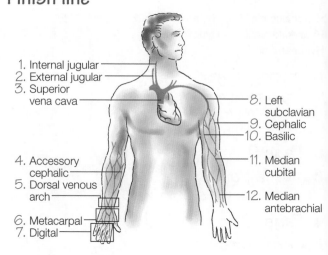

1. Internal jugular
2. External jugular
3. Superior vena cava
4. Accessory cephalic
5. Dorsal venous arch
6. Metacarpal
7. Digital
8. Left subclavian
9. Cephalic
10. Basilic
11. Median cubital
12. Median antebrachial

Match point

1. B, F, 2. C, D, F, 3. A, E, G

■ **Page 20**
Power stretch

Saline lock: C, D, E, H, I
Piggyback method: B, C, G
Volume-control set: A, F

Hit or miss

1. True.
2. False. There's no circumvented I.V. administration set.
3. True.
4. True.
5. False. I.V. tubing varies according to factors such as type of infusion and infusion contents.

■ **Page 21**
Finish line

1. Drops delivered by macrodrip (amount): 10, 15, or 20 gtt/minute

2. Drops delivered by microdrip (amount): 60 gtt/minute

3. Formula for calculating flow rate:

$$\frac{\text{vol of infusion (ml)}}{\text{time of infusion (min)}} \times \text{drop factor (gtt/ml)} = \text{flow rate (gtt/min)}$$

4. How to adjust to the calculated rate: After calculating the flow rate, remove your watch or position your wrist to look at your watch and the drops at the same time. Next, adjust the clamp to achieve the ordered flow rate and count the drops for 1 full minute. Readjust the clamp as necessary, and count drops for another minute. Keep adjusting the clamp and counting drops until you have the correct rate.

Page 22
Strikeout

1. Examples of commonly used infusion control devices include clamps, volumetric pumps, time tapes, ~~water seal chambers~~, and rate minders.
2. Factors that can affect the flow rate include the following: type of I.V. fluid, the viscosity of the I.V. fluid, the height of the infusion container, the type of administration set, the size and position of the venous access device, ~~and the number of venipuncture attempts~~.
3. Factors that can affect the flow rate when using a clamp include ~~number of hours of sleep~~, vein spasms, vein pressure changes, patient movement, manipulations of the clamp, and bent or kinked tubing.
4. Many nurses routinely check the flow rate whenever they're in a patient's room, ~~every 15 minutes~~, and after each position change.
5. More frequent flow rate checks are required for patients who are critically ill, who have conditions that might be exacerbated by fluid overload, ~~who complain of feeling cold~~, who are very young or elderly, or who are receiving drugs that can cause tissue damage if infiltration occurs.

Jumble gym

1. Ph lebit is
2. I nfi lt r a t ion
3. Circu lat ory overload
4. Adv e r s e drug r ea ctions

Answer: Heart failure

Page 23
Mind sprints

- Progress notes
- Computerized chart
- Special I.V. sheet or flow sheet
- Nursing care plan
- Intake and output sheet
- Medication sheet

Strikeout

5. ~~Time of patient's last meal and bowel movement~~
7. ~~Solution's manufacturer and expiration date~~
9. ~~List of potential interactions~~

Page 24
Hit or miss

1. True.
2. False. Input should be documented every 1 to 2 hours for children and critically ill patients.
3. True.
4. False. It's important to document all reasons for discontinuation.
5. False. Unused solution isn't considered output.

Jumble gym

1. Proced u re
2. Equ i pment
3. D i scomfort
4. A ctivity r est r iction s
5. T ra n s ient pai n
6. Cold s ensation

Answer: Stress reduction

Chapter 2
Page 27
Mind sprints

- Administering drugs, blood and blood products, and nutrients
- Maintaining hydration
- Restoring fluid and electrolyte balance
- Providing fluids for resuscitation
- Emergency or surgical procedures

Strikeout

4. ~~Depositing all used catheters and needles in a double-bagged trash bin in the patient's bathroom~~
7. ~~Checking the practitioner's orders and modifying them when necessary~~
10. ~~Teaching venipuncture to the nurse's aide~~
12. ~~Discontinuing all I.V. solutions at the end of every shift~~

Page 28
Strikeout

2. ~~Height~~
5. ~~Family history~~
6. ~~Last medication given~~
9. ~~Last hospitalization~~

Boxing match

2. Infiltration, 3. Hearing loss, 4. Bleeding, 5. Infection, 6. Heart damage

Page 29
Hit or miss

1. True. 2. False. Most use plastic containers. 3. True. 4. True. 5. True. 6. False. They remove pathogens and particles and prevent air from entering the veins. 7. True. 8. False. A more viscous solution produces larger drops and therefore requires a macrodrip system, which delivers fewer drops. 9. True. 10. True. 11. True. 12. False. They're primarily used for pediatric patients. 13. True.

Page 30
You make the call

1. Type of set: Volume-control (also called a *burette set* [or Buretrol])
   Uses: Primarily used for pediatric patients because it delivers small, precise amounts of fluid or medication from a volume-control chamber that's calibrated in milliliters
2. Type of set: Basic
   Uses: Most common type used to deliver an I.V. solution or to infuse solutions through an intermittent infusion device, the Y-site provides a secondary injection port for a separate or simultaneous infusion of two compatible solutions
3. Type of set: Add-a-line (also called a secondary set)
   Uses: Delivers an intermittent infusion through one or more additional Y-sites, or Y-ports

■ Page 31
Batter's box
1. C, 2. E, 3. A, 4. B, 5. D

Mind sprints
- Outdated solution (expired date on container)
- Cracks or chips (glass container), tears or leaks (plastic container)
- Cloudy, unclear, turbid, or separated solution
- Change of color (from known or usual color)
- Missing label on solution container

■ Page 32
Match point
1. B, 2. A, 3. C

■ Page 33
Hit or miss
1. False. They're routinely used and their use improves the safety and accuracy of drug and fluid administration.
2. True.
3. True.
4. False. The device should be disengaged, otherwise, medication will continue to infuse into the infiltrated area.

Starting lineup

Attach the pump to the I.V. pole, and then insert the administration spike into the I.V. container.

⬇

Fill the drip chamber completely to prevent air bubbles from entering the tubing, and clamp the tubing while the pump door is open.

⬇

Prime and place the I.V. tubing, making sure to flush all the air out of the tubing before connecting it to the patient.

⬇

Place the infusion pump on the same side of the bed as the I.V. setup and the intended venipuncture site.

⬇

Set the appropriate controls to the desired infusion rate or volume.

⬇

Check the patency of the venous access device, watch for infiltration, and monitor the accuracy of the infusion rate.

■ Page 34
Winner's circle

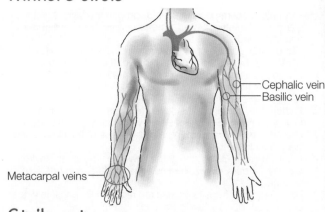

Cephalic vein
Basilic vein
Metacarpal veins

Strikeout
1. ~~Usually, the most prominent veins are the best choices.~~ These veins aren't necessarily the best veins because they're often sclerotic from previous use.
5. ~~You should try to select a vein in the patient's dominant arm or hand whenever possible.~~ You should select a vein from a nondominant arm or hand whenever possible.
6. ~~For subsequent venipunctures, you should select sites below the previously used or injured vein.~~ You should select sites above the previously used vein.

■ Page 35
Power stretch
Cephalic: B   **Basilic**: C
Digital: A, E   **Antecubital**: F, G
Metacarpal: D, H

Memory jogger
Vein
Infusion
Patient

■ Page 36
Hit or miss
1. False. The superficial veins in these sites are generally best.
2. True.
3. True.
4. False. The metacarpals are in the hand and the cephalic and basilic veins are most suitable for irritating drugs and solutions with a high osmolarity.
5. True.
6. True.
7. True.
8. False. It carries an increased risk of thrombophlebitis.
9. True.
10. True.

Batter's box
1. I or E, 2. I or E, 3. C, 4. B, 5. D, 6. J, 7. G, 8. F, 9. K, 10. A, 11. H

■ Page 37
Finish line

Layers of the skin

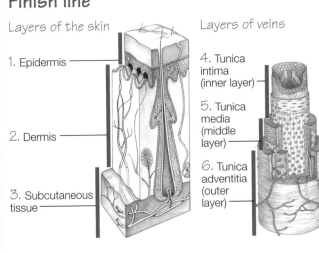

Layers of veins

1. Epidermis

2. Dermis

3. Subcutaneous tissue

4. Tunica intima (inner layer)

5. Tunica media (middle layer)

6. Tunica adventitia (outer layer)

■ Page 38
Power stretch

Tunica media: G, I

Dermis: F, J

Tunica adventitia: E, K

Epidermis: A, L

Subcutaneous tissue: H, C

Tunica intima: B, D

■ Page 39
Strikeout

1. ~~Time of day when venipuncture or infusion will occur~~
6. ~~Patient's blood type~~
7. ~~Patient's privacy~~

■ Page 40
Hit or miss

1. True.
2. True.
3. True.
4. True.
5. False. Most over-the-catheter needles are available in lengths of 1″ and 1¼″ ; longer needles are typically used in surgical procedures.
6. True.
7. False. Winged catheters have short, small-bore tubing, they're especially useful for hard veins and for intermittent or one-time-only use.
8. True.
9. False. Although commonly used for I.V. bolus injections, butterfly needles should be used when the patient is in stable condition, has adequate veins, and requires I.V. fluids or medications for only a short time.

■ Page 41
You make the call

1. *Type of device:* Over-the-needle catheter

   Purpose: Long-term therapy for the active or agitated patient

   Advantages: Inadvertent puncture of veins less likely than with winged needle set, more comfortable for patient, radiopaque thread for easy insertion, syringe (on some units) permits easy check of blood return and prevents air from entering vessel on insertion, rarely requires activity-restricting devices (such as armboards)

   Disadvantages: Difficult to insert, requires extra care during insertion

2. *Type of device:* Winged needle set

   Purpose: Short-term therapy (such as single-dose infusion) for cooperative patient, therapy for a neonate or child, or for an elderly patient with fragile or sclerotic veins

   Advantages: Easiest intravascular device to insert because the needle is thin-walled and very sharp, ideal for nonirritating I.V. push drugs.

   Disadvantages: Difficult to use with deep veins or obese patients.

■ Page 42
Match point

1. C, 2. B, 3. E, 4. A, 5. D

Mind sprints

- Size of the vein
- Health (tone) of the vein
- Osmolarity of drug or solution
- pH of drug or solution
- Concentration of solution
- Infusion rate

■ Page 43
Cross-training

						¹I		²A	R	M	³B	O	A	R	⁴D	
						O					U				U	
				⁵F		N					T				A	
				L		⁶S			T				L		
				A		S		O				T				L	
				S		L		P		⁷T	O	U	R	N	I	Q	U	E	T
				H		I		⁸L	H			F				M	
				B		N		U	O			L				E	
				A		E		E	R			Y				N	
⁹C	H	L	O	R	H	E	X	I	D	I	N	E				
				K		O		L	S			E				
						C		O	I			E		¹⁰P		
						K		C	S			D		O		
						K		¹¹N			L		V		
				¹²A	N	E	S	T	H	E	T	I	C		
						E					D				
						D					O				
¹³B	E	V	E	L				N				
				E		¹⁴G	A	U	G	E			

■ Page 44
Strikeout

1. A properly distended vein should appear and feel round, firm, and ~~partially filled with blood~~. It should also rebound when gently compressed.
2. Because the amount of trapped blood depends on circulation, a patient who's hypotensive, ~~overly hydrated~~, very cold, or experiencing vasomotor changes (as in septic shock) may have inadequate filling of the peripheral blood vessels.
3. If the patient's skin is cold, you should warm it by rubbing and stroking his arm; covering the entire arm with warm, moist towels for 5 to 10 minutes; ~~or applying a 10% menthol solution to the skin surface~~.
4. The ideal tourniquet is one that can be secured easily, ~~turns the skin beneath and around it purple~~, doesn't roll into a thin band, stays relatively flat, and releases easily.
5. A too-tight tourniquet can impede arterial blood flow, impede venous blood flow, cause bruising (especially in elderly patients whose veins are fragile), ~~cause an allergic reaction~~, and obliterate the radial pulse.

Starting lineup

Place the tourniquet under the patient's arm, about 6″ (15 cm) above the venipuncture site.
Place the arm on the middle of the tourniquet.
Bring the ends of the tourniquet together, placing one on top of the other.
Holding one end on top of the other, lift and stretch the tourniquet and tuck the top tail under the bottom tail—without loosening the tourniquet.
Tie the tourniquet smoothly and snugly, being careful not to pinch the patient's skin or pull his arm hair.

■ Page 45
Boxing match

1. Chlorhexidine, 2. Povidone-iodine, 3. Iodine, 4. Lidocaine, 5. Transdermal analgesic, 6. Iontophoresis, 7. Epinephrine

You make the call

Procedure: Injecting a local anesthetic.

Relevance: Injection of a local anesthetic (such as lidocaine) may be ordered when starting peripheral I.V. therapy. Lidocaine anesthetizes the site to pain while allowing the patient to feel touch and pressure.

■ Page 46
Strikeout

2. ~~Lidocaine is best administered directly into the vein, where it can take immediate effect~~. Lidocaine injected into the vein will cause systemic effects, it should be injected intradermally only for anesthetic effects.
6. ~~A lidocaine injection should keep the skin numb for at least 1 hour~~. This injection should keep the skin numb for about 30 minutes.

Batter's box

1. A, 2. E, 3. B, 4. I, 5. J, 6. G, 7. D, 8. C, 9. H, 10. F

■ Page 47
Match point

1. I, 2. D, 3. B, 4. H, 5. E, 6. G, 7. A, 8. F, 9. C

■ Page 48
Starting lineup

Grasp the plastic hub with your dominant hand and remove the cover.
Examine the device. If the edge isn't smooth, discard the device and obtain another one.
Tell the patient that you're about to insert the device, and ask him to remain still and refrain from pulling away.
Insert the device, bevel up, through the skin and into the vein at a 5- to 15-degree angle (deeper veins require a wider angle).
Lower the hub (the distal portion of the adapter) until it's almost parallel to the skin.
Advance the device to at least one-half its length, at which point you should see blood in the flashback chamber.

Hit or miss

1. False. This usually occurs only when a venous access device enters a thick-walled vein or when the patient has good tissue tone.
2. True.
3. False. Advancing the needle at this point can puncture the vein and therefore should be avoided.
4. True.
5. True.
6. False. You should advance the catheter only, and maintain a rapid flow rate to dilate the vein; advancing the needle could puncture the vein.
7. False. Although this technique reduces the risk of puncturing a vein, it increases the risk of infection.
8. True.
9. True.

■ Page 49
You make the call

Device: Male luer-lock adapter plug, also known as a *saline lock*

Reason for use: This device allows you to convert an existing I.V. line into an intermittent infusion device when venous access must be maintained for intermittent use and continuous infusion isn't necessary. It keeps the access device sterile and prevents blood and other fluids from leaking from an open end.

Mind sprints

- Maintains a keep-vein-open status
- Minimizes the risk of fluid overload and electrolyte imbalances
- Reduces the risk of contamination
- Lowers cost
- Allows greater patient mobility

■ Page 50
Train your brain

Answer: To ensure patency and prevent occlusion, flush the device before and after infusing medication.

Batter's box

1. A, 2. E, 3. B, 4. F, 5. D, 6. C

■ Page 51
Starting lineup

After putting on gloves, palpate the area with your fingertips until you feel the vein.
Clean the skin over the vein with a cleaning solution, swiping in a side-to-side motion.
Aim the device directly over the vein, and stretch the skin with your fingertips.
Insert the device about one-half to two-thirds its length at a 15-degree angle to the skin.
Look for blood in the flashback chamber.
Remove the tourniquet and inner needle, and advance the catheter.

Strikeout

1. ~~To collect blood, you'll need all of the following equipment: one or more evacuated tubes, a 26G needleless system, an appropriate-size syringe without a needle, and a protective pad.~~ You'll need a 19G needle, not a 26G needle to prevent hemolysis.
2. ~~You should leave the tourniquet tied until after the syringe is attached and the appropriate amount of blood is withdrawn.~~ Untie the tourniquet after the venipuncture to avoid damaging the vein with high pressure.
3. ~~You should wait 10 minutes after blood collection before attaching a saline lock or I.V. tubing, then regulate the flow rate and stabilize the device.~~ You should quickly attach the I.V. tubing after blood collection to prevent clotting.

■ Page 52
You make the call
1. Method: Chevron method

   Procedure: Cut a long strip of ½" tape and place it sticky-side-up under the hub. Cross the ends of the tape over the hub, and secure the tape to the skin on the opposite sides of the hub. Apply a piece of 1" tape across the wings of the chevron. Loop the tubing and secure it with another piece of tape.

2. Method: U method

   Procedure: Cut a strip of ½" tape. With the sticky side up, place it under the hub of the catheter. Bring each side of the tape up, folding it over the wings of the catheter. Press it down, parallel to the hub. Next apply tape to stabilize the catheter.

3. Method: H method

   Procedure: Cut three strips of ½" tape. Place one strip of tape over each wing, keeping the tape parallel to the catheter. Place the third strip of tape perpendicular to the first two. Then put tape directly on top of the wings, making sure the catheter is secure.

Hit or miss
1. True.
2. False. Standard methods are the chevron, H, and U methods.
3. False. Tape ends shouldn't meet, this can cause a tourniquet effect if infiltration occurs.
4. True.
5. False. Removing hair should be done with scissors or electric clippers to decrease microabrasions and risk of infection.
6. True.
7. False. Swelling and redness are signs of impending complications.
8. False. Paper tape shouldn't be used for dressings because it shreds and is difficult to remove after prolonged contact with skin and body heat.

■ Page 53
Mind sprints
- Avoids the need for daily dressing changes
- Causes fewer skin reactions
- Allows clear view of insertion site to check for complications (especially helpful in detecting early signs of phlebitis and infiltration)
- Is waterproof, protecting site from contamination if it gets wet
- Less likely to become dislodged because of good adherence

You make the call
Procedure: Applying a semipermeable dressing

Why it's done: A transparent, semipermeable dressing allows air to pass through but keeps the venous access site impervious to microorganisms, thereby preventing infection.

■ Page 54
Jumble gym
1. Stretch net
2. Arm board
3. Semipermeable transparent dressing
4. Flexion
5. Dislodgment
6. Immobilization

Answer: Range of motion

Mind sprints
- Date and time of venipuncture
- Number of the solution container (if required)
- Type and amount of solution
- Name and dosage of additives in solution
- Type of venipuncture device used (including length and gauge)
- Venipuncture site
- Number of venipuncture attempts (if more than one)
- Flow rate
- Adverse reactions and actions taken to correct them
- Patient teaching and evidence of patient understanding
- Name of person initiating infusion

■ Page 55
Batter's box
1. A, 2. D, 3. E, 4. B, 5. C, 6. F

Starting lineup

Wash your hands and put on sterile gloves.

Hold the catheter in place with your nondominant hand, then gently remove the tape and the dressing.

Assess the venipuncture site for signs of infection, infiltration, and thrombophlebitis.

If you detect any sign of complications, apply pressure to the area with a sterile gauze pad and remove the catheter or needle, maintain pressure until bleeding stops, and then apply an adhesive bandage. Using new equipment, insert the I.V. access at another site.

If you don't detect complications, hold the needle or catheter at the hub and carefully clean around the site with an alcohol swab or another approved solution. Allow the site to dry completely.

Retape the device and apply a transparent semipermeable dressing, or apply gauze and secure it.

(Note: The answer is still correct if the fourth and fifth steps are interchanged.)

■ Page 56

Strikeout

2. ~~To avoid microbial growth, you shouldn't allow an I.V. solution container to hang for more than 48 hours.~~ To avoid microbial growth, you shouldn't allow an I.V. solution container to hang for more than 24 hours.
4. ~~You should always preset the flow rate before spiking and hanging a new I.V. container to save time.~~ You should set the flow rate after spiking a new I.V. container.
5. ~~Most facilities dictate changing I.V. administration sets on a daily basis (for a primary infusion line) and whenever contamination is suspected.~~ Most facilities dictate changing I.V. administration sets every 96 hours.

Power stretch

Additive infusion: A, D

Vein dissection: B, C, E

■ Page 57

Hit or miss

1. False. They're embedded in fat, which makes them difficult to isolate.
2. True.
3. True.
4. False. The scalp has an abundant supply of veins, it's the most commonly used site for those under age 6 months.
5. True.
6. True.
7. False. An artery, not a vein, has a palpable pulse.
8. True.
9. False. Tourniquets shouldn't be used on infants. If a tourniquet effect is needed, you should tip the infant's head down to facilitate filling the superficial veins.
10. False. The preferred device is a small-diameter, winged over-the-needle catheter.
11. False. Avoid overtaping the I.V. site because it makes inspecting the site and surrounding tissue difficult and tape removal is particularly traumatic to the infant.
12. True.

Finish line

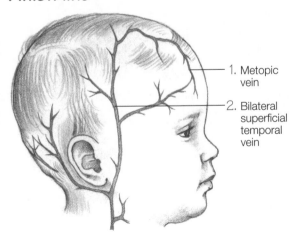

1. Metopic vein
2. Bilateral superficial temporal vein

■ Page 58

Strikeout

1. ~~Veins in elderly patients are typically not prominent and are more difficult to see.~~ The veins of these patients are typically more prominent than those of younger patients.
5. ~~It's best to perform a venipuncture slowly on an older patient to avoid excessive bruising.~~ It's best to perform a venipuncture quickly on an older patient to avoid bruising.
7. ~~You should keep the tourniquet on longer than usual with an elderly patient to ensure the vein stays distended during venipuncture.~~ You should remove a tourniquet from this patient promptly to prevent bleeding through the vein wall around the infusion device cause by increased vascular pressure.
9. ~~An elderly patient's veins also appear large if venous pressure is inadequate.~~ An elderly patient's veins appear large if venous pressure is adequate.

Team up!

Local
- Catheter dislodgment (extravasation)
- Cellulitis
- Hematoma
- Infiltration
- Nerve, tendon, or ligament damage
- Occlusion
- Phlebitis
- Severed or fractured catheter
- Thrombophlebitis
- Thrombosis
- Vasovagal reaction
- Vein irritation or pain at I.V. site
- Venous spasm

Systemic
- Allergic reaction
- Circulatory overload
- Embolism
- Septicemia

■ Page 59

Match point

1. D, 2. G, 3. M, 4. F, 5. C, 6. E, 7. N, 8. I, 9. O, 10. A, 11. K, 12. B, 13. H, 14. L, 15. J

■ Page 60
Mind sprints
- Signs and symptoms
- Patient's complaints
- Name of practitioner notified
- Treatment ordered and given

Starting lineup

After putting on gloves, lift the tape from the skin to expose the insertion site. Avoid manipulating the device to prevent organisms from entering the skin and to prevent discomfort.

▼

Apply a sterile 2″ × 2″ dressing directly over the insertion site, and then quickly remove the device.

▼

Maintain direct pressure on the site for several minutes, and then tape a dressing over it, being careful not to encircle the limb. If possible, hold the limb upright for about 5 minutes to decrease venous pressure.

▼

Tell the patient to restrict his activity for about 10 minutes and to leave the dressing in place for at least 8 hours. Advise him to apply warm, moist packs if tenderness lingers at the site.

▼

Dispose of used venipuncture equipment, tubing, and solution in the designated receptacles.

▼

Document the time of removal, the catheter length and integrity, and the condition of the site. Also record how the patient tolerated the procedure and any nursing interventions.

■■ Chapter 3
■ Page 64
Batter's box
1. A or C, 2. A or C, 3. B, 4. D, 5. G, 6. F, 7. E, 8. H

Strikeout
3. ~~Provides a way to draw arterial blood samples~~ This is a way to draw venous, not arterial, blood samples.
6. ~~Reduced risk of thrombus formation~~ The risk of thrombus formation increases.
8. ~~Reduces risk of sepsis~~ The risk of sepsis increases.

■ Page 65
Finish line

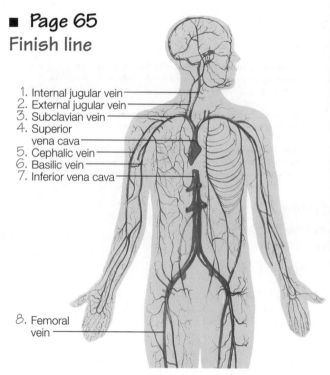

1. Internal jugular vein
2. External jugular vein
3. Subclavian vein
4. Superior vena cava
5. Cephalic vein
6. Basilic vein
7. Inferior vena cava
8. Femoral vein

Mind sprints

Life-threatening risks
- Pneumothorax
- Sepsis
- Thrombus formation
- Perforation of the vessel and adjacent organs

Catheter-related disadvantages
- Requires more time and skill to insert than a peripheral I.V. catheter
- Costs more to maintain than a peripheral I.V. catheter
- Carries a risk of air embolism

■ Page 66
Power stretch
Superior vena cava: A, C, D, F, G, H
Inferior vena cava: B, E, I

Hit or miss
1. False. About 5 L of blood circulate throughout the body.
2. True.
3. False. Circulation enters the right atrium, not ventricle.
4. True.
5. False. Blood flows rapidly in the venae cavae, at about 2,000 ml/minute.
6. True.
7. False. The access device would terminate in the superior vena cava.
8. True.

■ Page 67
Match point
1. C, 2. B, 3. A

■ Page 68

Jumble gym

1. Nontunneled catheter
2. Tunneled access device
3. Peripherally inserted central catheter
4. Implanted ports

Answer: Introducers

■ Page 69

You make the call

Catheter type: Tunneled CV access device

How it's inserted: The access device enters the subclavian vein and terminates in the superior vena cava; it's tunneled through the subcutaneous tissue to an exit site on the skin (usually located by the nipple); a Dacron cuff helps hold the access device in place.

Strikeout

2. ~~The silicone used in tunneled access deivces is less physiologically compatible than polyurethane or polyvinyl and, therefore, is more likely to cause thrombosis and irritation or damage to the vein lining.~~ Silicone is more physiologically compatible and, therefore, less likely to cause thrombosis and vein irritation or damage.

6. ~~Most cuffs used in tunneled access devices contain silver ions that provide antibacterial protection for about 3 months.~~ Most cuffs are made of Dacron; an alternate type contains silver ions that provide antibacterial protection for up to 3 months.

7. ~~Nontunneled access devices are changed every 5 days to prevent infection.~~ To avoid infection, nontunneled access devices are changed according to facility policy and usually whenever the injection site appears red; the optimal time for removing them is unknown.

■ Page 70

Mind sprints

Medications	Conditions
■ Antibiotics	■ Cancer
■ Chemotherapy	■ Acquired immunodeficiency syndrome
■ TPN	■ Intestinal malabsorption
■ Blood products	■ Anemia
	■ Organ transplants
	■ Bone or organ infections

Boxing match

1. Multilumen, 2. Groshong, 3. Hickman, 4. Broviac, 5. Long-line

■ Page 71

Batter's box

1. D, 2. J, 3. C, 4. H, 5. B, 6. G, 7. A, I, or F, 8. A, I, or F, 9. F, 10. E

Gear up!

☑ CV access device
☑ Extra syringes and blood sample containers (for venous samples, if ordered)
☑ Heparin or saline flush solution
☐ Implantable pump
☑ Infusion pump
☑ Linen-saver pad
☑ Local anesthetic
☑ 3-ml syringe with 25G needle (for introduction of anesthetic)
☑ Antimicrobial solution
☑ Scissors
☑ Sterile dressing
☑ Sterile gauze pads
☑ Sterile mask, gown, and gloves
☑ Sterile syringe (for blood samples)
☑ Sterile towels or drapes
☑ Suture material
☐ Tuberculin syringe
☐ Implanted port
☐ Warming blanket

■ Page 72

Hit or miss

1. False. Not all PICCs have guide wires.
2. True.
3. False. Tuberculin and 3-ml syringes should be avoided because they create too much pressure in the PICC line and can cause it to burst; a 10-ml syringe should be used instead.
4. False. In many states, registered nurses who are specially trained and skilled in the proper insertion technique are permitted to insert PICCs; PICCs are inserted at the bedside, whereas tunneled access devices are surgically inserted.
5. False. This type of catheter is a midline catheter; it isn't a true CV access device because its tip terminates in the axillary vein, not in the inferior or superior vena cava.
6. True.
7. False. A PICC may be unsuitable for someone with bruising, scarring, or sclerosis from earlier venipunctures; it works best when introduced early in treatment and shouldn't be used as a last resort.
8. True.
9. True.
10. False. All catheters, regardless of composition, should be checked frequently for signs of phlebitis and thrombus formation.

■ Page 73
Finish line

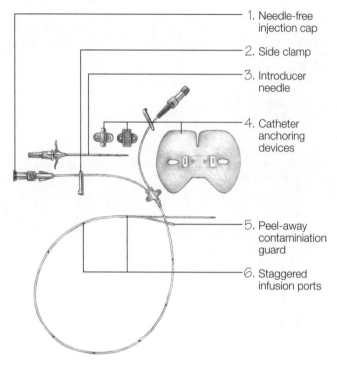

1. Needle-free injection cap
2. Side clamp
3. Introducer needle
4. Catheter anchoring devices
5. Peel-away contaminiation guard
6. Staggered infusion ports

Memory jogger

S = Saline
A = Additive
S = Saline
H = Heparin

■ Page 74
Strikeout

4. ~~The implanted port is commonly threaded through either the femoral vein at the shoulder or the common ileal vein at the base of the neck.~~ It's commonly threaded through the subclavian vein at the shoulder or through the jugular vein at the base of the neck.
6. ~~Using an implanted port for self-infusion of medication is comfortable and extremely convenient for the patient.~~ Because the patient must insert a special needle through subcutaneous tissue to access an implanted port, daily infusions are both uncomfortable and inconvenient.

Mind sprints

- Easier to maintain than external devices
- Require heparinization only once per month to maintain patency
- Pose less risk of infection
- Pose fewer activity restrictions
- Require fewer self-care measures and dressing changes

■ Page 75
Batter's box

1. F, 2. G, 3. A, 4. B, 5. E, 6. D, 7. C

Finish line

Top view

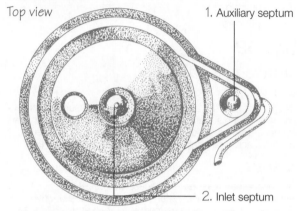

1. Auxiliary septum
2. Inlet septum

Cross-sectional view

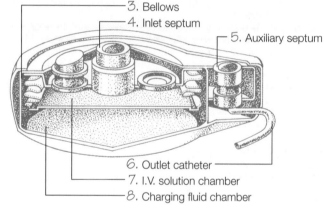

3. Bellows
4. Inlet septum
5. Auxiliary septum
6. Outlet catheter
7. I.V. solution chamber
8. Charging fluid chamber

■ Page 76
Mind sprints

- Type of access device
- Patient's anatomy and age
- Duration of therapy
- Vessel integrity and accessibility
- History of previous neck or chest surgery such as mastectomy
- Presence of chest trauma
- Possible complications

Power stretch

Internal jugular: B, E, J, K
Basilic: C, G, L
Subclavian: A, F, H, L, M
External jugular: D, N, B, K
Cephalic: C, I, L

Page 77

Strikeout

2. ~~Insertion of an access device in the femoral vein is usually less difficult in a larger patient.~~ Insertion is more difficult in a larger patient.
4. ~~The femoral vein site inherently carries a lower risk of local infection than other veins.~~ It carries a higher risk of infection because of the difficulty of keeping a dressing clean and intact in the groin area.
5. ~~When a femoral vein is used in CV therapy, the patient's leg needs to be kept straight; however, movement isn't generally limited.~~ Movement should be limited to prevent bleeding and to keep the access device from becoming dislodged; also, infection can occur at the insertion site from the access device's moving into and out of the incision.

Jumble gym

1. Punctured carotid artery
2. Uncontrolled hemorrhage
3. Emboli
4. Impeded blood flow

Answer: Brain damage

Page 78

Cross-training

Mind sprints

- Presence of scar tissue
- Interference with surgical site or other therapy
- Configuration of lung apices
- Patient's lifestyle or daily activities

Page 79

Hit or miss

1. True.
2. False. The patient will be placed in Trendelenburg's position, with his head lowered and his body and legs inclined.
3. True.
4. False. A venogram may be ordered beforehand to check the status of vessels; afterward, blood samples are drawn to establish baseline coagulation levels, and a chest X-ray is taken to confirm access device placement.

Batter's box

1. C, 2. F, 3. G, 4. B, 5. H, 6. A, 7. D, 8. E

Page 80

Starting lineup

> Attach the tubing to the solution container.

> Prime the tubing with the solution.

> Fill the syringes with saline or heparin flush solutions, based on facility policy and procedure.

> Prime and calibrate any pressure monitoring setups.

> Recheck all connections to make sure they're secure.

> Cover all open ends of the access device with sealed caps.

You make the call

Position: Trendelenburg's position

Why it's used: It's used for insertion of a CV access device into the subclavian or internal jugular vein. This position distends the neck and thoracic veins, making them more visible and accessible. Filling the veins also lessens the chance of air emboli because venous pressure is higher than atmospheric pressure.

Page 81

Batter's box

1. E, 2. F, 3. A, 4. H, 5. J, 6. I, 7. G, 8. C, 9. B, 10. D

■ Page 82
Starting lineup

Place a linen-saver pad under the site to prevent soiling.

↓

Clip the patient's hair from around the site to prevent infection from microorganisms.

↓

Swab the site with chlorhexidine using a back-and-forth motion.

↓

Adjust sterile drapes to uncover the patient's eyes, if necessary.

Strikeout

3. ~~In many cases, the nurse is asked to perform fluoroscopy and inject contrast dye to assist with access device placement.~~ Nurses don't perform fluoroscopy; this is handled by the doctor and radiology department.
6. ~~Whenever the access device hub is open to air, such as when changing syringes during blood sampling, the nurse must tell the patient to take a deep breath to make sure there is enough air in the line.~~ The nurse tells the patient to perform Valsalva's maneuver or clamps the port to decrease the risk of air embolism.
9. ~~Elevating the head of the patient's bed 45 degrees after applying the dressing will ensure that the infusion flows by gravity.~~ Elevating the head of the bed helps the patient to breathe more easily.

■ Page 83
Match point
1. C, 2. B, 3. A

Memory jogger
Clamp
Clean
Connect

Mind sprints
- Difficulty with changing the access device
- Difficulty with maintaining an occlusive dressing
- Kinking of the access device

■ Page 84
Starting lineup

Clean the site with chlorhexidine using the same method as the initial skin preparation.

↓

Cover the site with a transparent semipermeable dressing.

↓

Seal the dressing with nonporous tape, checking that all edges are well secured.

↓

Label the dressing with the date and time, your initials, and the catheter length.

Mind sprints
- Type of access device used
- Location of insertion
- Access device tip position (as confirmed by X-ray)
- Patient's tolerance of the procedure
- Blood samples taken

■ Page 85
Batter's box
1. F, 2. K, 3. I, 4. G, 5. J, 6. D, 7. C, 8. H, 9. B, 10. A, 11. E

Gear up!
- ☑ Chlorhexidine swabs
- ☑ Clean gloves
- ☐ Irrigation solution
- ☐ Local anesthetic for injection
- ☑ Sterile drape
- ☑ Sterile gloves and masks
- ☐ Sutures
- ☐ Syringe
- ☑ Transparent semipermeable dressing

■ Page 86
In the ballpark
Dressing: Every 4 to 7 days
Solution: Every 24 hours
Tubing: Every 72 hours
Caps: Every 7 days

Photo finish
1. Removing the old dressing
2. Cleaning the insertion site
3. Redressing the site

■ Page 87

Mind sprints

- Redness
- Swelling
- Tenderness
- Drainage

Starting lineup

| Wash your hands, and then place the patient in a comfortable position. |

▼

| Prepare a sterile field. Open the bag, placing it away from the sterile field, but within reach. |

▼

| Put on clean gloves and remove the old dressing. |

▼

| Inspect the old dressing for signs of infection. Culture discharge at the site or on the old dressing (if needed), and dispose of the old dressing and gloves in the bag. |

▼

| Check the position of the access device and the insertion site for infiltration or infection. |

▼

| Put on sterile gloves, and clean the skin around the access device with chlorhexidine using a back-and-forth or side-to-side motion. |

▼

| Redress the site with a transparent semipermeable dressing. |

▼

| Label the dressing with the date, time, and your initials. |

▼

| Discard all used items properly, then reposition the patient comfortably. |

■ Page 88

Hit or miss

1. False. You don't need to wear a mask unless there's a contamination risk.
2. False. The INS recommends changing the solution every 24 hours and the tubing every 72 hours.
3. True.
4. True.
5. False. Because higher heparin concentrations can interfere with the patient's clotting factors, the lowest concentration should be used.
6. True.
7. True.
8. True.
9. False. Always use strict aseptic technique when changing the cap.
10. True.

Strikeout

Step 3: ~~If multiple infusions are running, wait until only one infusion is left running before stopping the infusion to collect the blood sample.~~ If multiple infusions are running, stop them and wait 1 minute before drawing blood; this allows enough time for fluids and medications to be carried from the access device, preventing them from mixing with the sample being collected.

Step 4: ~~Clean the end of the injection cap with heparin solution.~~ Caps are cleaned with an antiseptic swab.

Step 5: ~~Place a 5-ml lavender-top evacuated tube into its plastic sleeve, and use this tube to collect and discard the filling volume of the access device, plus and extra 5 to 10 ml of blood.~~ It's only necessary to collect an extra 2 to 3 ml of blood.

Step 8: ~~Failure to get blood to flow from the access device using the above technique means that the access device is completely occluded; the only alternative is to use a syringe to obtain the blood sample.~~ If you can't get blood flowing from the access device, the tip of the access device might be against a vessel wall. Try having the patient raise his arms over his head, turn on his side, cough, or perform Valsalva's maneuver, or flush the catheter with saline solution before making another attempt to draw blood.

■ Page 89

Power stretch

Kinked access device: C, E, G, H
Fibrin sheath: A, D, H
Disconnected access device: B, I
Access device tear: F, J, K

Match point

1. A, 2. C, 3. B

■ Page 90
Cross-training

Crossword solution:

			¹A			²F	I	S	T	U	³L	A	
			I		⁴H	E					O		
			R		E						C		
		⁵P	N	E	U	M	O	T	H	O	R	A	X
			M		O						L		
			B		T						I		
	⁶C	H	Y	L	O	T	H	O	R	A	X	N	
	Y		L		O						F		
	D		I		R						E		
	R		S		A		⁸S				C		
	O		M		X		E				T		
	T						P				I		
	H		⁹S	E	P	T	I	C	S	H	O	C	K
	O						I				N		
¹⁰T	H	R	O	M	B	O	S	I	S		S		
	A												
	X												

■ Page 91
Mind sprints
- Chest pain
- Dyspnea
- Cyanosis
- Decreased or absent breath sounds on the affected side

Memory jogger
ACT:

Acute respiratory distress,

Chest wall motion that's asymmetrical,

Tracheal shifting away from the affected side

Match point
1. B, 2. A, 3. D, 4. E, 5. C

■ Page 92
Batter's box
1. K, 2. E, 3. G, 4. F, 5. B, 6. I, 7. A, 8. H, 9. D, 10. C, 11. J

Match point
1. B, 2. C, 3. F, 4. A, 5. E, 6. D

■ Page 93
Strikeout

Step 3: ~~Explain the procedure to the patient, and tell him that he'll be instructed to take a deep breath as the access device is withdrawn.~~ The patient should be instructed to perform Valsalva's maneuver, not take a deep breath, to prevent air embolism during withdrawal of the access device.

Step 5: ~~Position the patient sitting upright on the edge of the bed.~~ The patient should be positioned supine to prevent emboli.

Step 7: ~~Stop infusing all medications, but maintain a saline infusion to keep the vein open.~~ All infusions should be stopped.

Starting lineup

Clip the sutures and remove the access device in a slow, even motion as the patient performs Valsalva's maneuver.

↓

Apply antimicrobial ointment to the insertion site to seal it.

↓

Inspect the access device to see if any pieces broke off during the removal. If so, notify the practitioner immediately and monitor the patient closely for signs of distress.

↓

Place a transparent semipermeable dressing over the site, and label the dressing with the date and time of removal and your initials.

↓

Properly dispose of the I.V. tubing and equipment you used.

↓

Continue to monitor the patient and the insertion site frequently for the next few hours for evidence of air emboli and insidious bleeding.

■ Page 94
Hit or miss
1. True.
2. False. Common implantation sites include the arm, chest, abdomen, flank of the chest, or thigh.
3. True.
4. False. It reduces the number of venipunctures.
5. True.
6. True.
7. False. Noncoring needles, not conventional needles, are used.

You make the call
Type of implanted port: Top-entry implanted port

How it's accessed: With this type of port, the most commonly used, the needle is inserted perpendicular to the reservoir.

■ Page 95
Three-point conversion

1. **Straight noncoring needle**: Only type of needle used with a side-entry port; may also be used to access a deeply implanted top-entry port
2. **Right-angle noncoring needle**: Most common type of noncoring needle; allows for perpendicular insertion into a top-entry port
3. **Right-angle noncoring needle with extension set**: Used when administering a bolus injection or continuous infusion; can be easily secured to the patient

Starting lineup

A small incision is made, and the catheter is introduced into the superior vena cava through the subclavian, jugular, or cephalic vein.

↓

Fluoroscopy is used to verify placement of the catheter tip.

↓

A subcutaneous pocket is made over a bony prominence on the chest wall, and the catheter is tunneled to the pocket.

↓

The catheter is connected to the port reservoir, which is placed in the pocket and flushed with heparinized saline solution.

↓

The reservoir is sutured to the underlying fascia, and the incision is closed.

↓

A dressing is applied to the wound site.

■ Page 96
Boxing match

2. Venogram, 3. Informed consent, 4. Prophylactic, 5. Infiltration, 6. Heparinization

■ Page 97
Mind sprints

- Infection
- Clotting
- Redness
- Device rotation or port housing movement
- Skin irritation

Starting lineup

Attach the tubing to the solution container.

↓

Prime the tubing with fluid.

↓

If setting up an intermittent system, fill two syringes— one with 10 ml of normal saline solution and the other with 5 ml of heparin solution (100 units/ml).

↓

Prime the noncoring needle and extension set with saline solution from the syringe. (Prime the tubing and purge it of air using strict aseptic technique.)

↓

After priming the tubing, recheck all connections for tightness. Make sure that all open ends are covered with sealed caps.

■ Page 98
Hit or miss

1. True.
2. True.
3. True.
4. False. These are signs and symptoms of sepsis. Infiltration causes swelling, tenderness and, possibly, burning or stinging at the site.
5. True.

Starting lineup

With the patient sitting upright and with his back supported, palpate the area over the port to locate the septum.

⬇

Anchor the port between your thumb and the first two fingers of your nondominant hand. Then, using your dominant hand, aim the needle at the center of the device, between your thumb and first finger.

⬇

Insert the needle perpendicular to the port septum. Push the needle through the skin and septum until you reach the bottom of the reservoir (you'll feel the back of the port).

⬇

Check the needle placement by aspirating for a blood return.

⬇

If you can't obtain blood, remove the needle and repeat the procedure. If you still can't obtain a blood return, notify the practitioner immediately.

⬇

Flush the device with normal saline solution. If you detect swelling or the patient complains of pain, remove the needle and notify the practitioner.

■ Page 99
Mind sprints

- Hemorrhage, trauma, or surgery within past 10 days
- Active internal bleeding
- Intracranial neoplasm
- Hypersensitivity to thrombolytic agents
- Liver disease
- Stroke in the past 2 months
- Subacute bacterial endocarditis
- Visceral tumors

Starting lineup

Palpate the area over the port, and then access the implanted port.

⬇

Check for a blood return.

⬇

Flush the port with 5 ml of saline solution, and clamp the extension tubing.

⬇

Attach the syringe containing the prescribed thrombolytic agent and unclamp the extension tubing.

⬇

Instill the thrombolytic using a gentle pull-push motion on the syringe plunger to mix the solution in the access equipment, port, and catheter.

⬇

Clamp the extension set, and leave the solution in place for 15 minutes (up to 30 minutes in some facilities).

⬇

Attach an empty 10-ml syringe, unclamp the extension set, and aspirate the thrombolytic and clot with the 10-ml syringe; then discard the syringe. If the clot can't be aspirated, wait 15 minutes before trying again.

⬇

After the blockage is cleared, flush the catheter with at least 10 ml of saline solution, and then flush with heparin solution.

■ Page 100
Match point
1. C, 2. D, 3. A, 4. E, 5. B

Starting lineup

> Gather the necessary equipment: a 10-ml syringe filled with 5 ml of normal saline solution, a 10-ml syringe filled with 5 ml of sterile heparin flush solution (100 units/ml), sterile gloves, sterile 2″ × 2″ gauze pad, and tape.

> After shutting off the infusion, clamp the extension set and remove the I.V. tubing.

> Attach the syringe filled with saline solution using aseptic technique.

> Unclamp the extension set, flush the device with saline solution, and remove the saline solution syringe.

> Attach the heparin syringe, flush the port with the heparin solution, and clamp the extension set.

> Remove the noncoring needle, and dispose of it properly.

> Document the procedure and your findings.

■ Page 101
Jumble gym
1. **S**kin infec**ti**on
2. Skin **b**reak**do**wn
3. Extrava**s**ation
4. Fi**br**in s**h**ea**t**h for**m**ation

Answer: Thrombosis

Starting lineup

> Put on gloves.

> Place the gloved index and middle fingers from the nondominant hand on either side of the port septum.

> Stabilize the port by pressing down with the index and middle fingers, maintaining pressure until the needle is removed.

> Using your gloved, dominant hand, grasp the noncoring needle and pull it straight out of the port.

> Apply a dressing as indicated.

> If no more infusions are scheduled, remind the patient that he'll need a heparin flush in 4 weeks.

■ Page 102
Batter's box
1. D, 2. C, 3. K, 4. H, 5. E, 6. B, 7. A, 8. G, 9. I, 10. J, 11. F, 12. L

■ Chapter 4
■ Page 105
Mind sprints
- I.V. bolus injection
- Intermittent infusion
- Continuous infusion

Batter's box
1. H, 2. C, 3. D, 4. B, 5. E, 6. F, 7. G, 8. A

■ Page 106
Hit or miss

1. False. One of the major benefits of the I.V. route is the ability to administer drugs while the patient is unconscious.
2. True.
3. True.
4. False. Drugs given subQ or I.M. are absorbed erratically because muscle and skin can delay drug passage, drugs given I.V. are absorbed very quickly.
5. True.
6. True.
7. False. Accurate titration involves adjusting the concentration and administration rate of the infusate.
8. False. Dilution requires a larger, not smaller, volume of solute.

Train your brain

Answer: Administering a drug I.V. and not orally avoids first-pass metabolism by the liver.

■ Page 107
Power stretch

Physical: B, H, D, E, G
Chemical: A, B, C, F, H
Therapeutic: B, H, I

Strikeout

2. ~~Very few I.V. drugs are compatible with commonly used I.V. solutions.~~ Most I.V. drugs are compatible with commonly used I.V. solutions.
3. ~~The more complex the solution, the less risk exists for incompatibility.~~ The more complex the solution, the greater the risk of incompatibility.
4. ~~An I.V. solution containing divalent cations (such as calcium) has a lower incidence of incompatibility.~~ A solution containing divalent cations such as calcium increases the risk of incompatibility.

■ Page 108
Match point

1. B, 2. E, 3. D, 4. A, 5. F, 6. C

Boxing match

1. Vasoconstriction, 2. Hypovolemia, 3. Repeated venipunctures, 4. Irritating

■ Page 109
Jumble gym

1. Hypersensitivity
2. Idiosyncratic reaction
3. Anaphylaxis
4. Cross-sensitivity

Answer: Preservatives

■ Page 110
Mind sprints

- The patient's weight in kilograms
- The patient's body surface area (BSA)

Hit or miss

1. False. To convert from pounds to kilograms, divide by 2.2.
2. True.
3. True.
4. False. Adding an I.V. drug requires recalculating the original infusion rate to accommodate the needed changes.

■ Page 111
You make the call

Calculation tool: Nomogram for adult patients
Calculation tool: Nomogram for pediatric patients

How they're used: Find the patient's weight in the right column and his height in the left column. Mark these two points, and then draw a line between them. The point where the line intersects the surface area in the center gives you the patient's BSA in square meters (m^2). If the patient is a child of average size, you can determine BSA from weight alone by using the shaded area.

■ Page 112
Batter's box

1. E, 2. H, 3. D, 4. C, 5. G, 6. F, 7. A, 8. B

Strikeout

1. ~~You should always maintain clean technique when administering I.V. medications.~~ Always maintain aseptic technique.
4. ~~When drawing up a drug before adding it to the primary solution, you should always use two syringes.~~ You should use one syringe that's large enough to hold the entire dose.

■ Page 113
Team colors

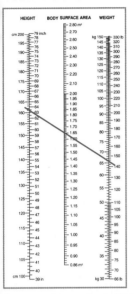

Answer: The patient's BSA is 1.912 m².

■ Page 114
Match point
1. C, 2. E, 3. A, 4. D, 5. B

Hit or miss
1. False. Always check the expiration date on all drugs and diluents before use.
2. True.
3. True.
4. False. After reconstitution, it's important to check the admixture for evidence of incompatibilities.
5. False. Most drugs are moderately acidic, it's important to know this because incompatibility is more likely with drugs or I.V. solutions that have a high or low pH.
6. True.

■ Page 115
Starting lineup

Draw up the amount and type of diluent specified by the manufacturer.

Clean the rubber stopper of the drug vial with an alcohol swab, using aseptic technique.

Connect the syringe to the needleless adapter on the vial.

Inject the diluent into the drug vial.

Mix the solution by gently rotating the vial.

Watch to ensure that the powder is thoroughly dissolved. If it isn't fully dissolved, let the vial stand for 10 to 30 minutes, if necessary, agitate it several times gently to dissolve the drug.

Check for visible signs of incompatibility once the drug is fully reconstituted.

Mind sprints
- Single-dose ampules or vials
- Multidose vials
- Prefilled syringes
- Disposable cartridges

■ Page 116
Starting lineup

Adding to an I.V. bottle

> Clean the rubber stopper or latex diaphragm with alcohol.

> Attach the needleless adapter and the medication-filled syringe into the center of the stopper or diaphragm, and inject the drug.

> Invert the bottle at least twice to ensure thorough mixing.

> Remove the latex diaphragm, and insert the administration spike.

Adding to a plastic I.V. bag

> Attach the needleless adapter and the medication-filled syringe into the clean latex medication port.

> Inject the drug.

> Grasp the top and bottom of the bag, and quickly invert it twice.

Adding to an infusing I.V. solution bag

> Make sure the primary solution container has enough solution to provide adequate dilution.

> Clamp the I.V. tubing, and take down the container.

> Clean the rubber injection port with an alcohol swab.

> Inject the drug, keeping the container upright.

■ Page 117
Match point

1. C, 2. B, 3. A, 4. D, 5. H, 6. F, 7. E, 8. G

You make the call

Type of equipment: Needleless system

Describe the highlighted areas: The blunt-tipped insertion device and rubber injection port are known as *access*, or *adaptation*, devices. The insertion device allows you to piggyback drugs or additional I.V. solutions without the use of a needle, thereby greatly reducing the risk of accidental needle stick injuries. The port has a pre-established slit that can open and reseal immediately, it may be used as part of a special administration set or an adapter for an existing set.

■ Page 118
Memory jogger

- Right drug
- Right patient
- Right time
- Right dosage
- Right route

Hit or miss

1. True.
2. True.
3. False. Emergency drugs must be given rapidly to provide an immediate effect.
4. False. Such patients may require a slower injection time or more highly diluted drugs to avoid decreased drug intolerance.

■ Page 119
Finish line

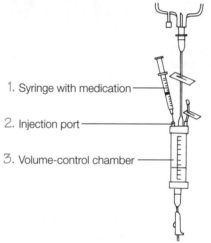

1. Syringe with medication
2. Injection port
3. Volume-control chamber

Power stretch

Piggyback method: B, F, G
Saline lock: A, E, F, G, I, J
Volume-control set: C, D, H

■ Page 120
Batter's box

1. C, 2. F, 3. D, 4. A, 5. E, 6. B

■ Page 121
Finish line

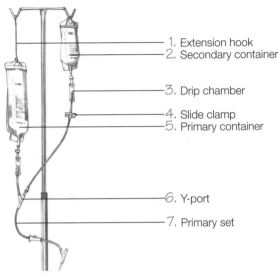

1. Extension hook
2. Secondary container
3. Drip chamber
4. Slide clamp
5. Primary container
6. Y-port
7. Primary set

■ Page 122
Starting lineup

> Attach the minibag to the administration set, and prime the tubing with the drug solution.

> Secure a needleless device to the I.V. tubing, and prime the device with the drug solution.

> Clean the cap on the saline lock with an alcohol swab.

> Stabilize the saline lock with the thumb and index finger of your nondominant hand.

> Insert the needleless device of a syringe containing flush solution into the center of the injection cap, then pull back the plunger slightly to watch for a blood return, and slowly inject the flush solution.

> Insert the needleless device attached to the administration set into the saline lock.

> Regulate the drip rate, and infuse the medication as ordered.

You make the call

Answer: The nurse is stabilizing the saline lock with her thumb and index finger to prevent movement at the insertion site while preparing to insert a needleless device containing saline flush solution into the lock's cap. Stabilization is necessary because any movement increases the risk of phlebitis and catheter dislodgment.

■ Page 123
Hit or miss

1. True.
2. False. You shouldn't write directly on the chamber because the plastic can absorb ink. Instead, you should place a label on the chamber, taking care not to cover the numbers on the chamber.
3. False. The chamber should be gently rotated to mix the medication and solution, vigorous shaking may dislodge the device or cause air bubbles or a spill.
4. True.
5. True.
6. True.

Starting lineup

> Fill the chamber with 20 ml of fluid.

> Open the flow-regulating clamp.

> Squeeze and hold the drip chamber.

> Close the regulating clamp directly below the drip chamber.

> Release the drip chamber.

■ Page 124
Boxing match

1. Loading dose, 2. Insulin, 3. Fluid overload, 4. Electrolyte levels

Batter's box

1. A, 2. E, 3. F, 4. C, 5. I, 6. D, 7. H, 8. B or G, 9. B or G

■ Page 125
Match point

1. B, 2. F, 3. G, 4. A, 5. C, 6. D, 7. E

Hit or miss

1. False. Drug dosage is based on the child's weight, each patient has a different normal dosing.
2. True.
3. False. The most common method of delivering I.V. medications to children is by intermittent infusion, using a volume-control set.
4. True.
5. True.
6. False. Watch for signs of respiratory depression or CNS depression, including confusion, when giving an I.V. analgesic to an elderly patient.

■ Page 126
Cross-training

	¹S				²R											
³H	Y	P	E	R	S	E	N	S	I	T	I	V	I	T	Y	
	S				S											
	T			⁴P	H	L	E	B	I	T	I	S				
	E				I						⁵T		⁶A			
	M				R						O		N			
⁷C	I	R	C	U	L	A	T	O	R	Y	O	V	E	R	L	O	A	D
	C				T						E		P			
	I				O						R		H			
⁸I	N	F	I	L	T	R	A	T	I	O	N		A			
	F				Y								X			
	E				D		⁹S				C		I			
	C				E		P				E		A			
	T				P		E						X			
	I				R		¹⁰V	E	N	O	U	S	S	P	A	S	M
	O				E		D									
	N				S		S									
					S		H									
					I		O									
¹¹R	E	N	A	L	T	O	X	I	C	I	T	Y				
					N		K									

■ Page 127
Match point
1. C, 2. B, 3. E, 4. A, 5. D

Strikeout
2. ~~Phlebitis can follow any infusion, but it's more common after a direct injection of medication.~~ It's more common after continuous infusions.
3. ~~Phlebitis develops more rapidly in larger veins that are closer to the heart.~~ Phlebitis develops more rapidly in distal veins than in those closer to the heart.
7. ~~Applying ice to the affected area can ease the patient's discomfort.~~ To ease discomfort, apply warm packs, or soak the arm in warm water.

■ Page 128
Jumble gym
1. **D**elayed healing
2. **T**issue necrosis
3. **E**xtravasation
4. **D**isfigurement
5. **A**mputation

Answer: Vesicant drugs

Hit or miss
1. False. To avoid tendon and nerve damage, avoid using the back of the hand, the wrist and fingers are difficult to immobilize and should also be avoided.
2. False. Infusions should be started with dextrose 5% in water or normal saline solution.
3. True.
4. True.
5. True.

■ Chapter 5
■ Page 131
Cross-training

					¹C	O	A	G	U	L	A	T	I	²O	N
		³T			R									X	
⁴E	R	Y	T	H	R	O	C	Y	⁵T	E	S			Y	
		A			S			H						G	
		N		⁶F	S		R						E	
		S		L	M		O			⁷R		N	
		F		U		⁸A	N	E	M	I	A		H	
		U		I		T		B				F		⁹P
		S		D		C		O		¹⁰L		A		L
		I		V		H		C		E	C		¹¹A	B	O
		O		O		I		Y		U	T		S	
		N		L		N		T		K	O		M	
				U		G		¹²H	E	M	O	R	R	H	A	G	E
				M				S		C	S			
				E						Y				
					¹³H	E	M	O	L	Y	T	I	C	
										E				
										S				

■ Page 132
Batter's box
1. B, 2. E, 3. D, 4. G, 5. A, 6. F, 7. C

Power stretch
Fluid volume: C, F, L
Oxygen-carrying capacity: A, D, H, I, J, B, F
Coagulation capacity: B, E, F, G, K, M

Page 133

Strikeout

3. ~~Peripheral veins are used for acute transfusions because of their larger diameters and ability to deliver large volumes of blood quickly.~~ Central veins are best used for acute transfusions because of their larger diameters and ability to deliver large volumes of blood quickly.

4. ~~A 24-gauge peripheral I.V. catheter is commonly used for transfusions.~~ A 20-gauge or larger peripheral catheter is commonly used.

7. ~~Because transfusion therapy carries few risks and provides great benefits, the patient's consent is unnecessary.~~ The patient must be informed of the risks of a transfusion; many facilities have special consent forms for the procedure.

Mind sprints

- Gloves
- Mask
- Goggles
- Gown

Page 134

Match point

1. E, 2. B, 3. D, 4. C, 5. A

Finish line

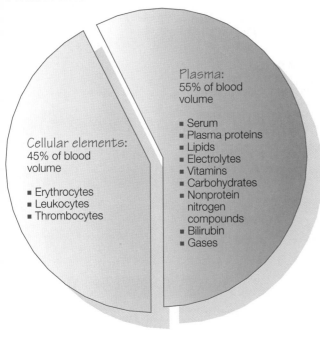

Plasma:
55% of blood volume

- Serum
- Plasma proteins
- Lipids
- Electrolytes
- Vitamins
- Carbohydrates
- Nonprotein nitrogen compounds
- Bilirubin
- Gases

Cellular elements:
45% of blood volume

- Erythrocytes
- Leukocytes
- Thrombocytes

Page 135

Mind sprints

- ABO typing
- Rh typing
- Crossmatching
- Direct antiglobulin test
- Antibody screening test
- Screening for such diseases as hepatitis B and C, HIV, human T-cell lymphotrophic virus type 1 (HTLV-1) and type II (HTLV-2, or hairy cell leukemia), syphilis, and cytomegalovirus

Hit or miss

1. True.
2. False. It destroys RBCs and may be life-threatening.
3. True.
4. True.
5. False. Each blood group is named for a specific antigen, not antibody.
6. True.
7. False. The naturally occurring antibodies are anti-A and anti-B.
8. True.
9. False. Such major antigens are inherited.
10. True.

Page 136

Jumble gym

1. Un**i**versal bl**oo**d **d**onor
2. Universal bl**oo**d rec**i**p**i**ent
3. Imm**u**nogeni**c**
4. **H**uman leukoc**y**te ant**i**gens

Answer: Hemolytic

Page 137

Strikeout

3. ~~Rh-negative blood contains a variant of the D antigen or D factor.~~ This variant is found in Rh-positive blood.

5. ~~A serious hemolytic reaction typically follows the first exposure to Rh-positive blood in a person who is Rh-negative.~~ The first exposure won't cause a reaction because anti-Rh antibodies are slow to form; however, subsequent exposures may pose a risk of hemolysis and agglutination.

7. ~~Most people in the United States have Rh-negative blood.~~ Only about 10% of the U.S. population has Rh-negative blood.

You make the call

Answer: During her first pregnancy, an Rh-negative woman becomes sensitized to Rh-positive fetal blood factors due to placental blood exchange, but her antibodies usually aren't sufficient to harm the fetus. In a subsequent pregnancy with an Rh-positive fetus, increasing amounts of the mother's anti-Rh antibodies attack the fetus, destroying RBCs. This can cause various problems for the neonate (including jaundice, liver problems, even brain damage) and can lead to life-threatening hemolytic disease in severely affected infants if not treated soon after delivery.

■ Page 138
Circuit training

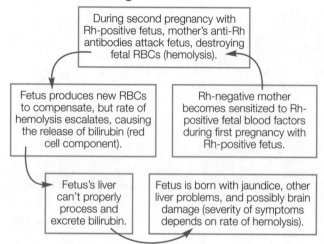

Batter's box

1. D, 2. E, 3. B, 4. A, 5. C, 6. I, 7. F, 8. G or K, 9. G or K, 10. J, 11. H

■ Page 139
Power stretch

Autologous: B, D, E

Homologous: A, C

Strikeout

1. ~~Donors must be at least 21 and weigh at least 132 lb (60 kg) to give blood.~~ Donors must be at least 17 and weigh at least 110 lb (50 kg).
2. ~~Those with acquired immunodeficiency syndrome (AIDS) can donate blood as long as they are presently taking three HIV drugs and strictly adhere to their medication regimen.~~ Anyone diagnosed with HIV or AIDS is ineligible to donate, regardless of medication regimen.
5. ~~Those who have received tattoos within the past 5 years can't donate blood.~~ Those who have been tattooed within the past 12 months are ineligible to donate.

■ Page 140
Memory jogger

Check: informed consent, personal identification, ABO and Rh status, blood bank identification number, and expiration date

Verify: all information with another nurse or doctor, following facility protocol

Inspect: blood for abnormalities

Power stretch

Whole blood: D, H

Packed red blood cells: A, G

Platelets: C, E

Fresh frozen plasma: B, F

■ Page 141
Hit or miss

1. False. Packed RBCs consist of blood from which 80% of the plasma has been removed.
2. False. Whole blood and packed RBCs begin to deteriorate after 4 hours at room temperature; they should be ordered just before a transfusion.
3. True.
4. True.
5. False. Platelets are used to control bleeding; granulocytes are used to fight antibiotic-resistant septicemia and other life-threatening infections.
6. True.

Boxing match

1. Leukocyte removal filter, 2. Cell washing, 3. Centrifuge, 4. Sedimentary agents

■ Page 142
Gear up!

☑ Blood component to be transfused
☑ Blood warmer, if ordered
☐ Dextrose 5% in water
☐ Foley catheter
☑ Gloves
☑ Goggles
☑ Gown
☑ Infusion pump, if ordered
☑ In-line or add-on filter
☑ I.V. pole
☑ Mask
☐ N.G. tube
☑ Normal saline solution
☑ Pressure cuff, if needed
☑ Sphygmomanometer
☑ Venipuncture equipment
☐ Warfarin

Match point

1. B, 2. A, 3. C

■ Page 143
Mind sprints

- Abnormal color
- Clumping of RBCs
- Gas bubbles
- Presence of extraneous material (possibly indicates bacterial contamination)

Starting lineup

Gather a Y-type blood administration set, an I.V. pole, and a venous access device.

▼

Close all the clamps on the I.V. administration set.

▼

Insert the spike of the line you're using for the normal saline solution into the saline solution bag.

▼

Open the port on the blood bag, and insert the spike of the line you're using to administer the blood or blood component into the port.

▼

Hang both bags on the I.V. pole.

▼

Open the clamp on the line of normal saline solution, and squeeze the drip chamber until it's half full of normal saline solution.

▼

Remove the adapter cover at the tip of the blood administration set, open the main flow clamp, and prime the tubing with normal saline solution; close the clamp and recap the adapter.

▼

Attach the blood administration set to the venous access device using a needleless connection, and flush it with the normal saline solution.

■ Page 144
Finish line

Blood group	Compatible RBCs
Recipient	
O	**O**
A	**O, A**
B	B, O
AB	**A, A, B, O**
Donor	
O	O, A, B, AB
A	**A, AB**
B	B, AB
AB	**AB**

Strikeout

3. ~~Generally, a transfusion is run at a fast flow rate of 85 gtt/minute for the first 10 to 30 minutes.~~ Transfusions are generally run at a slow rate—usually 20 gtt/minute—for the first 10 to 30 minutes to observe for transfusion reactions.
5. ~~Platelets and coagulation factors may be given more slowly than RBCs and granulocytes.~~ They may be administered at a faster rate than RBCs and granulocytes.
6. ~~A transfusion shouldn't take more than 8 hours.~~ No transfusion should take longer than 4 hours; the risk of contamination and sepsis increases after that.
7. ~~Any unused blood following a transfusion can be resealed and stored on the nursing unit for future emergency use.~~ Unused blood should be discarded or returned to the blood bank.
8. ~~It's extremely important to monitor the patient's vital signs every 10 minutes throughout the transfusion.~~ Vital signs are usually monitored every 15 minutes for the first hour, then according to the patient's transfusion history and facility policy for the remainder of the transfusion.

▪ Page 145
Mind sprints

- Fever
- Chills
- Rigors (shaking)
- Headache
- Nausea
- Facial flushing
- Respiratory distress (wheezing, dyspnea, bronchospasm)
- Itching

Starting lineup

Quickly clamp the blood infusion line to stop the transfusion; don't dispose of the blood bag.

▼

Reestablish the normal saline infusion (if using a straight-line infusion); if using a Y-set, use a new bag of saline solution and tubing.

Check and record the patient's vital signs.

▼

Notify the practitioner.

▼

Continue to observe the patient; if no additional signs of a reaction appear within 15 minutes, adjust the flow clamp to achieve the ordered infusion rate, as ordered.

▼

Monitor the patient throughout the entire transfusion.

▪ Page 146
You make the call

Device: Pressure cuff

Why it's used: A pressure cuff may be used to increase the transfusion flow rate when rapid blood replacement is necessary. The cuff is placed over the blood bag like a sleeve and inflated, exerting uniform compression against all parts of the container. A pressure gauge, calibrated in millimeters of mercury (mm Hg), is attached to monitor the pressure.

▪ Page 147
Starting lineup

Prepare the patient, and set up the equipment as you would with a straight-line blood administration set.

▼

Prime the filter and tubing with normal saline solution to remove all air from the administration set.

▼

Connect the tubing to the needle or catheter hub.

▼

Insert your hand into the top of the pressure cuff sleeve, and pull the blood bag through the center opening; hang the blood bag loop on the hook provided with the sleeve.

▼

Hang the pressure cuff and blood bag on the I.V. pole; open the flow clamp on the tubing.

▼

Set the flow rate by turning the screw clamp on the pressure cuff counterclockwise; compress the pressure bulb of the cuff to inflate the bag to the desired flow rate. Then turn the screw clamp clockwise to maintain this constant rate.

Hit or miss

1. True.
2. False. Increasing the pressure increases the rate at which transfusion complications can develop.
3. False. Pressure should not exceed 300 mm Hg; excessively high pressure can cause hemolysis and damage the component container or rupture the blood bag.
4. True.

▪ Page 148
Batter's box

1. G, 2. B, 3. H, 4. D, 5. C, 6. A, 7. F, 8. E

▪ Page 149
Power stretch

Cryoprecipitate: B, F
Factor VIII: D, H
Albumin: A, C
Immune globulin: E, G

▪ Page 150
Train your brain

Answer: Never use a microaggregate filter to infuse platelets or plasma.

Match point

1. B, 2. C, 3. A

■ Page 151
Strikeout

2. ~~You should always use a 24- to 26-gauge venous access device to transfuse fresh frozen plasma in an emergency.~~ Fresh frozen plasma is given rapidly in an emergency and, therefore, requires a 20-gauge or larger venous access device.
3. ~~Large-volume transfusions of fresh frozen plasma may require correction for hypercalcemia.~~ The citric acid in fresh frozen plasma binds calcium, which causes hypocalcemia.
4. ~~Cross-typing is always necessary when administering albumin.~~ Cross-typing isn't necessary; in fact, albumin can be used as a volume expander in an emergency until crossmatching for whole blood is complete.
6. ~~You should always administer factor VIII concentrate slowly to prevent a hemolytic reaction.~~ Factor VIII concentrate is usually administered as rapidly as possibly to control bleeding; however, levels shouldn't exceed 6 ml/hour.
8. ~~Cryoprecipitate and factor VIII are essentially the same.~~ Cryoprecipitate contains fibrinogen, von Willebrand factor, factor XIII, and fibronectin in addition to factor VIII.
9. ~~Factor IX, or *antihemophilic factor,* is commonly used to treat hemophilia A.~~ Factor IX, or *Christmas factor,* is used to treat hemophilia B; hemophilia A is treated with factor VIII, or *antihemophilic factor.*
10. ~~Plasma products typically have a cloudy or turbid appearance.~~ Cloudiness or turbidity aren't normal; they could be an indication of contamination.

Batter's box

1. B, 2. E, 3. F, 4. I, 5. A, 6. D, 7. G, 8. H, 9. C

■ Page 152
In the ballpark

	Adults			Children		
Total blood volume	2.5 L	(5 L)	8 L	(75 ml/kg)	100 ml/kg	125 ml/kg
Prepared blood units	1/2 unit	(1 unit)	2 units	(1/2 unit)	1 unit	2 units
Catheter size	(20 gauge)	24 gauge	28 gauge	18 gauge	20 gauge	(24 gauge)

Hit or miss

1. True.
2. True.
3. False. The proportion of blood volume to body weight decreases as a child ages.
4. False. Older children should be told about the procedure, the purpose, and complications of a transfusion, using age-appropriate language.
5. True.
6. False. Older patients with preexisting heart disease may experience shortness of breath and other symptoms of heart failure when 1 unit of blood is transfused rapidly; they may be better able to tolerate half-unit transfusions.
7. False. Elderly patients tend to have a higher risk of delayed reactions and more severe reactions when they occur.
8. False. Elderly patients are less resistant to infection.

■ Page 153
Starting lineup

Stop the infusion.

Remove the catheter.

Cap the tubing with a new needleless connection.

Notify the practitioner.

Prepare to ice the site. (The site is usually iced for 24 hours, then warm compresses are applied.)

Document your observations and actions.

Promote reabsorption of the hematoma by having the patient gently exercise the affected limb.

Strikeout

1. ~~Check that the container is at least 12″ (30.5 cm) above the level of the I.V. site.~~ The container should hang at least 3′ (1 m) above the level of the I.V. site.
4. ~~Check to see if any blood cells have settled to the bottom of the bag; if so, the blood must be replaced.~~ Gently rock the bag back and forth to agitate any blood cells that may have settled on the bottom.

■ Page 154
Jumble gym

1. Acut**e** hemol**y**tic r**e**action
2. F**e**b**ri**le reaction
3. Alle**r**gic reaction
4. **P**lasma protein in**c**ompati**bi**lity
5. Bac**t**er**i**al **c**ontamination

Answer: Antipyretic

Mind sprints

- Fever
- Chills
- Headache
- Nausea
- Vomiting
- Hypotension
- Chest pain
- Dyspnea
- Nonproductive cough
- Malaise

■ Page 155

Match point

1. B, 2. C, 3. A, 4. D

Hit or miss

1. True.
2. False. Acute hemolytic reactions are life-threatening; they develop quickly and can lead to shock and renal failure.
3. True.
4. True.
5. False. Bacterial contamination most commonly involves gram-negative bacteria.
6. True.
7. False. Gas, clots, and a dark purple color may indicate bacterial contamination.

■ Page 156

Boxing match

1. Epinephrine, 2. Diuretic, 3. Vasopressor, 4. Antipyretic, 5. Antihistamine, 6. Broad-spectrum antibiotic

NCLEX reps

2. Allergic reactions may occur when the recipient reacts to allergens in the donor's blood; this reaction causes urticaria, flushing, and wheezing. A febrile reaction can occur, causing fever and urticaria, but it isn't accompanied by a rash. Diaphoresis, hot flashes, disorientation, and abdominal pain aren't symptoms of a transfusion reaction.

■ Page 157

Cross-training

¹A			²H										³F		
M			Y		⁴H	Y	P	O	⁵C	A	L	C	E	M	I	A
M			P						I			B				⁶H
O			O						R			R	⁷P			E
N			T			⁸B	A	C	T	E	R	I	A	L		M
I			H						U			L	A			O
⁹A	L	L	E	R	G	I	C		L			E	S			S
			R						A			R	M			I
			M	¹⁰P					T			E	A			D
			I	O					O			A	P			E
¹¹H		¹²A	N	T	I	P	Y	R	E	T	I	C	R			R
E			A	S			Y		T			T	O			O
M			S	S			O		I			I	T			S
O							V		O			O	E			I
¹³B	L	E	E	D	I	N	G	T	E	N	D	E	N	C	I	E	S
Y			U				R						N			
T			M				L									
I							O									
C		¹⁴O	X	Y	G	E	N	A	F	F	I	N	I	T	Y
							D									

■ Page 158

Hit or miss

1. False. Although all blood products are laboratory-tested and potential donors are carefully screened, neither precaution is foolproof; infectious diseases can still be transmitted through a transfusion.
2. False. Infectious diseases transmitted during a transfusion can go undetected for days, weeks, or months later, when signs and symptoms appear.
3. False. Most cases of posttransfusion hepatitis involve hepatitis C (non-A, non-B).
4. False. The test for hepatitis C isn't foolproof; it may yield false-negative results, allowing some cases to go undetected.
5. True.
6. True.
7. False. Most facilities test for CMV.
8. True.
9. False. All blood is routinely tested for syphilis.
10. False. Cold, not heat, kills off syphilis; the routine practice of refrigerating blood kills the organism, virtually eliminating the risk of contracting transfusion-related syphilis.

■ Chapter 6

■ Page 161

Batter's box

1. J or L, 2. J or L, 3. F or G, 4. F or G, 5. O, 6. A, 7. M, 8. C, 9. E, 10. D or H, 11. D or H, 12. B, 13. P, 14. K, 15. I or N, 16. I or N

■ Page 162

Power stretch

Cell cycle–specific: A, D, F
Cell cycle–nonspecific: B, C, E

Finish line

1. G_2 phase
2. M phase
3. G_0 phase
4. G_1 phase
5. S phase

■ Page 163
Mind sprints
■ The maximum safe dosage of a single drug wouldn't be enough to kill large numbers of cancerous cells; combining the drugs potentiates the effect, and the tumor responds as it would to a larger dose of a single drug.
■ Different drugs work at different stages of the cell cycle or by different mechanisms; using several drugs decreases the likelihood that the tumor will develop resistance to the chemotherapy.

Strikeout
2. ~~Generally, the drugs chosen for the first round of chemotherapy are the least effective.~~ The drugs given in the first round are usually the most effective because this is when cancer cells respond best to chemotherapy.
4. ~~A single course of chemotherapy involves administering one dose of a single drug.~~ A single course of chemotherapy involves giving repeated doses of a drug or a complement of drugs on a cyclic basis—daily, weekly, every other week, or every 3 to 4 weeks.
6. ~~Most patients require six treatment cycles before they show any beneficial response.~~ Although every patient differs, most show a beneficial response after three treatment cycles.

■ Page 164
Team up!
Cell cycle–specific drugs: Antimetabolites, Enzymes, Plant alkaloids

Cell cycle–nonspecific drugs: Alkylating agents, Antibiotic antineoplastics, Antineoplastics, Miscellaneous, Nitrosureas

Boxing match
1. Steroids, 2. Hormones, 3. Antihormones

■ Page 165
Power stretch
Antimetabolites: C

Plant alkaloids: F

Enzymes: B

Alkylating agents: D

Antibiotic antineoplastics: H

Hormones and hormone inhibitors: G

Folic acid analogs: A

Cytoprotective agents: E

■ Page 166
Hit or miss
1. True.
2. False. The drugs used in cancer immunotherapy are known as *biological response modifiers*.
3. True.
4. True.

Batter's box
1. F, 2. C, 3. B, 4. A, 5. E, 6. D

■ Page 167
Jumble gym
1. Interleukins
2. Colony-stimulating factors
3. Interferon alpha
4. Tumor necrosis factor

Answer: Messenger

■ Page 168
Strikeout
2. ~~The major sources of chemotherapy guidelines include the American Medical Association, the Centers for Disease Control and Prevention, and the International System of Units.~~ The major sources of chemotherapy guidelines include the American Society of Health-System Pharmacists, the Occupational Safety and Health Administration (OSHA), the Oncology Nursing Society, and the Infusion Nurses Society.

Mind sprints
■ Trained nurse
■ Pharmacist
■ Supervised pharmacy technician

■ Page 169
You make the call
1. Class II biological safety cabinet
2. Protective respirator

Why they're used: All chemotherapeutic drugs should be prepared in a well-ventilated workspace, such as a Class II biological safety cabinet or a vertical laminar airflow hood with a high-efficiency particulate air filter, which is vented to the outside to pull drug particles away from the drug compounder. If a Class II biological safety cabinet isn't available, OSHA recommends wearing a special respirator when mixing drugs.

Memory jogger
Gown (cuffed)

Gloves

Goggles (or face shield)

Gear up!
☑ 20G needles
☑ 70% alcohol
☑ Alcohol pads
☑ Appropriate diluent (if necessary)
☑ Chemotherapy gloves
☑ Chemotherapy spill kit
☐ Extension tubing
☑ Face shield or goggles and face mask
☑ Hazardous waste container
☑ Hydrophobic filter or dispensing pin
☐ Infusion pump
☐ I.V. containers and tubing
☐ I.V. pole
☑ Long-sleeved gown
☑ Medication labels
☑ Patient's medication order or record
☐ Patient-controlled analgesia pump
☐ Plasma and whole blood
☑ Plastic bags with "hazardous drug" labels
☑ Prescribed drugs
☑ Sharps container
☑ Sterile gauze pads
☑ Syringes with luer-lock fittings
☐ Tourniquet
☐ Venipuncture device

■ **Page 170**

Hit or miss

1. False. Gowns should be disposable, water resistant, and lint-free with long sleeves, knitted cuffs, and a closed front.
2. True.
3. False. Gloves should be powder-free because powder can carry contamination from the drugs into the surrounding air.
4. False. Double gloving is an option when the gloves aren't of the best quality.
5. True.
6. False. You should always wash your hands before putting on gloves and after removing them to prevent any inadvertent contamination from microbes or contact with toxic substances.
7. True.

Strikeout

1. ~~You should use a clean cloth and a mild soap detergent to clean the work surface of the safety cabinet before preparing drugs and after any spills.~~ You should use a sterile 70% alcohol solution and a disposable towel to clean surface areas and wipe up spills.
3. ~~If a drug comes in contact with your eye, you should immediately flood the eye with isopropyl alcohol while holding the eyelid open.~~ You should flood your eye immediately only with water or isotonic eyewash solution for at least 5 minutes.
8. ~~You should avoid using syringes and I.V. sets with luer-lock fittings; these can be difficult to remove and may cause a spill.~~ Luer-lock devices should be used with chemotherapeutic drugs because they are tight fitting and help prevent spills.
9. ~~You should always recap needles before putting them in a sharps container.~~ Recapping a needle can break the needle or puncture the skin.

■ **Page 171**

Boxing match

1. Shoe covers, 2. Respirator mask, 3. Goggles, 4. Powder-free gloves, 5. Dustpan, 6. Dessicant powder, 7. Cytotoxic

■ **Page 172**

Starting lineup

Put on protective garments, if you aren't already wearing them.

▼

Isolate the area and contain the spill with absorbent materials from the spill kit.

▼

Use the disposable dustpan and scraper to collect broken glass or dessicant absorbing powder.

▼

Carefully place the dustpan, scraper, and collected spill in a leakproof, puncture-proof, chemotherapy-designated hazardous waste container.

▼

Clean the spill area with a detergent or bleach solution.

■ **Page 173**

Batter's box

1. D, 2. C, 3. H, 4. G, 5. B, 6. E, 7. A, 8. F

■ **Page 174**

Power stretch

Vesicants: B, F

Nonvesicants: C, E

Irritants: A, D

■ **Page 175**

Hit or miss

1. True.
2. False. An extravasation kit is necessary when administering a vesicant drug.
3. False. A venous access device with the smallest possible gauge should be used to accommodate therapy and reduce the risk of infiltration.
4. True.
5. False. A low-pressure infusion pump should be used to administer vesicants through a peripheral vein to decrease the risk of extravasation.
6. True.
7. True.

You make the call

Equipment: Extravasation kit. Includes two pairs of gloves (surgical and protective for handling vesicants), syringes, cannulas, gauze pads, gauze dressings, adhesive tape, hot/cold pack, and antidotes (hyaluronidase and dimethylsulfoxide)

Why it's needed: Leakage of a vesicant solution into surrounding tissue is considered a medical emergency because it can cause tissue necrosis and sloughing. This kit contains all the supplies necessary to deal with an extravasation quickly.

■ **Page 176**

Strikeout

2. ~~Because chemotherapeutic drugs are so caustic, you should only select a vein that's hard and rigid.~~ You should select veins that are soft and pliable; hard, rigid veins are likely sclerosed and too difficult to access.
5. ~~Arms with functioning arteriovenous shunts, grafts, or fistulas for dialysis are obviously strong and therefore good candidates for chemotherapy infusions.~~ These limbs are compromised and unsuitable for chemotherapy.
6. ~~To avoid damage to the superficial nerves and tendons, you should use veins in the antecubital fossa and the back of the hand.~~ These veins should be avoided because they are too close to painful nerve centers.

■ Page 177
Starting lineup

Dispose of all needles and contaminated sharps in the red sharps container.

Dispose of unused medications, considered hazardous waste, according to your facility's policy.

Dispose of personal protective gear, glasses, and gloves in the yellow chemotherapy waste container.

Wash your hands thoroughly with soap and water, even though you have worn gloves.

Document the following: sequence in which drugs were administered; site accessed, gauge and length of catheter, and number of attempts; name, dose, and route of administered drugs; type and volume of I.V. solutions; and any adverse reactions and nursing interventions.

Put on protective clothing when handling the patient's body fluids for 48 hours after treatment.

Mind sprints

- Infiltration
- Extravasation
- Vein flare reactions

■ Page 178
Jumble gym

1. Compartment syndrome
2. Blisters
3. Vein thrombosis
4. Loss of consciousness
5. Stomatitis
6. Myelosuppression

Answer: Alopecia

■ Page 179
Hit or miss

1. True.
2. False. Organ system dysfunction and secondary malignancy are considered long-term effects of chemotherapy. Short-term effects include nausea and vomiting, alopecia, diarrhea, myelosuppression, and stomatitis.
3. True.
4. False. Hypersensitivity reactions can also occur with subsequent infusion of a drug.
5. False. Signs of extravasation include swelling, pain, and blanching (all similar to those of infiltration); respiratory distress, pruritus, chest pain, dizziness, and agitation are signs of acute hypersensitivity.
6. True.
7. False. Alopecia may affect the loss of all body hair.
8. True.
9. True.
10. False. These are signs of thrombocytopenia.

Batter's box

1. C, 2. F, 3. G, 4. D, 5. A, 6. E, 7. B

■ Page 180
Match point

1. I, 2. G, 3. A, 4. F, 5. D, 6. B, 7. H, 8. E, 9. K, 10. J, 11. C

■ Chapter 7
■ Page 183
Boxing match

1. Hyperalimentation, 2. Kilocalories, 3. Metabolism, 4. Gastrointestinal, 5. Central venous access

Strikeout

4. ~~A person's caloric requirements depend only on his amount of physical activity.~~ Caloric requirements are based on the individual's size, age, and sex in addition to physical activity.
5. ~~Parenteral solutions can only provide up to one-half of a person's daily nutritional requirements; the rest must come from solid food for metabolism to take place.~~ Parenteral nutrition can provide all of the body's nutritional and caloric needs to meet metabolic demands.
6. ~~PPN solutions generally provide more nonprotein calories than TPN solutions.~~ Generally these solutions provide fewer nonprotein calories than TPN because lower dextrose concentrations are used.

■ Page 184
Cross-training

	¹P									²H							
³A	L	B	U	M	I	N				Y		⁴P	⁵P	N			
R										P			R		⁶V		
A							⁷M	E	T	A	B	O	L	I	C		
L							R						T		T		
⁸H	Y	P	E	R	G	L	Y	C	E	M	I	A		E		A	
I		⁹H	Y	P	O	K	A	L	E	M	I	A		I		M	
C						M			¹⁰M		N		I		N	
I					E		A		¹¹D		S			
¹²A	L	I	M	E	N	T	A	R	Y	C	A	N	A	L		E	
E					T		N		X				
U		¹³L			A	U	¹⁴T	P	N		
S		I			T	T	R		
		P			I	R	O		
	¹⁵K	I	L	O	C	A	L	O	R	I	E	S		
	D			N	T	E		
	S			I		
			O		
	¹⁶S	U	B	C	L	A	V	I	A	N	

■ Page 185
Mind sprints

- Dextrose
- Proteins
- Lipids
- Electrolytes
- Vitamins
- Trace elements
- Water

Hit or miss

1. True.
2. False. Complications include catheter infection, hyperglycemia, and hypokalemia.
3. True.
4. True.
5. False. Parenteral infusions are given at a slow rate; central venous access device is necessary with infusions containing a dextrose concentration of 10% or higher because such solutions can cause vein sclerosis.
6. False. Parenteral nutrition is more expensive than enteral feedings.

■ Page 186
Power stretch

Peripheral parenteral nutrition: C, H, I, J
Total parenteral nutrition: A, B, D, E, F, G, K, L, M

■ Page 187
Batter's box

1. J, 2. G, 3. F, 4. E, 5. I, 6. H, 7. C, 8. D, 9. B, 10. A, 11. K

Circuit training

The body draws energy from the fats stored in adipose tissue.	→	The body taps its store of essential visceral proteins (serum albumin and transferrin) and somatic body proteins (skeletal, smooth muscle, and tissue proteins). These proteins and their amino acids are converted to glucose for energy through a process called *gluconeogenesis*.
↑		
The body mobilizes and converts glycogen to glucose through a process called *glycogenolysis*.		

■ Page 188
Mind sprints

- Cancer
- GI disorders
- Chronic heart failure
- Alcoholism
- Any condition that causes high metabolic needs (burns)

Power stretch

Marasmus: D, G, H
Iatrogenic: B, E, I
Kwashiorkor: A, C, F

■ Page 189
Strikeout

1. ~~You can obtain all the information you need for a thorough nutritional assessment based on the information in a patient's dietary history.~~ A thorough nutritional assessment includes obtaining a dietary history, performing a physical assessment, taking anthropometric measurements, and reviewing the results of pertinent diagnostic tests.
4. ~~The most commonly used anthropometric measurements include the patient's food preferences, personal habits, cultural influences, and religious beliefs.~~ Anthropometric measurements are objective measures of the patient's overall body size, composition, and specific body parts and include height, weight, ideal body weight, and body frame size.

■ Page 190
Match point

1. G, 2. E, 3. A, 4. F, 5. B, 6. H, 7. D, 8. I, 9. J, 10. C

■ Page 191

Jumble gym

1. Amino acids
2. Electrolytes and minerals
3. Micronutrients
4. Dextrose

Answer: Insulin

Mind sprints

- Sepsis
- Stress
- Shock
- Liver or kidney failure
- Diabetes
- Age
- Pancreatic disease
- Concurrent use of certain medications, including steroids

■ Page 192

Hit or miss

1. True.
2. True.
3. True.
4. False. Abruptly stopping a TPN solution can cause rebound hypoglycemia, not hyperglycemia.
5. False. TPN solutions are hypertonic, with an osmolarity of 1,800 to 2,600 mOsm/L.
6. False. TPN infusions may not be effective in severely stressed patients.
7. True.
8. True.

Match point

1. D, 2. E, 3. G, 4. B, 5. J, 6. C, 7. L, 8. K, 9. A, 10. H, 11. I, 12. F

■ Page 193

Mind sprints

- Sepsis
- Stress
- Shock
- Liver or kidney failure
- Diabetes
- Age
- Pancreatic disease
- Concurrent use of certain medications, including steroids

Strikeout

4. ~~PPN solutions are usually more concentrated than TPN solutions and therefore require less fluid.~~ PPN solutions are less concentrated than TPN solutions; therefore, they require more fluid to deliver nutrients.
5. ~~PPN is best reserved for patients with severe malnutrition or problems with fat metabolism.~~ PPN shouldn't be used for patients with moderate to severe malnutrition or fat metabolism disorders, such as pathologic hyperlipidemia, lipid nephrosis, and acute pancreatitis caused by hyperlipidemia.

■ Page 194

Power stretch

Continuous delivery: B, C, F

Cyclic therapy: A, D, E

Gear up!

- ☑ Alcohol swabs
- ☐ Blood collection kit
- ☑ Clean gloves
- ☐ Goggles
- ☐ Heparin solution
- ☑ Infusion pump
- ☑ I.V. administration set (with filtered tubing)
- ☑ I.V. pole
- ☐ Mask
- ☑ Practitioner's order
- ☑ Prescribed TPN solution
- ☐ Sterile dressings, tape
- ☐ Stethoscope
- ☐ Syringe
- ☐ Thermometer
- ☐ Venipuncture device
- ☐ Warming blanket

■ Page 195

Hit or miss

1. True.
2. False. A tunneled central venous access device, such as a Hickman, Broviac, or Groshong, may be used to administer long-term TPN therapy as well.
3. True.
4. False. The Food and Drug Administration requires the use of filters to deliver TPN.
5. False. Infusion of a chilled solution can cause discomfort, hypothermia, venous spasm, or venous constriction; the TPN container should be removed from the refrigerator about 1 hour before hanging it to allow for warming.
6. True.
7. True.
8. False. TPN solutions may hang for up to 24 hours.
9. False. You should maintain the flow rate as prescribed, even if the flow falls behind schedule.
10. False. You should never add medications to the TPN container.

Match point

1. D, 2. A, 3. B, 4. C

■ Page 196

Power stretch

Vital signs: A, C

Fingerstick test: E

Intake and output: A, D, G, H

Laboratory tests: B, F, G

Page 197

Strikeout

3. ~~"A gradual increase in flow rate is necessary to allow the pancreas to adjust to the increased glucose production needed because of the high level of insulin in the treatment."~~ The flow rate is increased gradually to allow the pancreas to establish and maintain the increased insulin production necessary to tolerate the treatment's high glucose content.

5. ~~"There are very tiny amounts of vitamins and minerals in TPN, so it isn't necessary to look for signs of deficiencies or toxicities."~~ Any abnormal level is significant and can cause serious patient problems; patients should be taught to look for signs and symptoms of vitamin and trace element deficiencies and toxicities.

6. ~~"TPN isn't really a medication, so you don't need to be concerned with incompatibility problems with other drugs."~~ TPN is considered a medication; therefore, the nurse should review all prescribed medications and over-the-counter preparations with the patient to check for incompatibilities.

Mind sprints

- Expiration date
- Time at which the solution was hung
- Glucose concentration
- Total volume of solution

Page 198

Cross-training

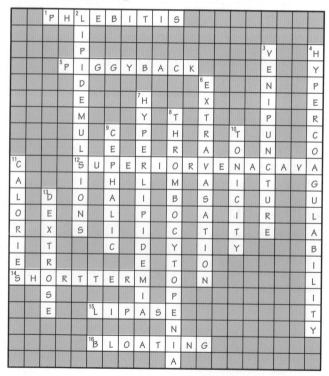

Page 199

Starting lineup

| Begin administering the continuous infusion. |
| Reduce the flow rate by one-half for 1 hour before stopping the infusion. |
| Stop the infusion. |
| Draw a blood glucose sample 1 hour after the infusion ends. |
| Observe for signs of hypoglycemia. |

Strikeout

2. ~~Adverse reactions occur in about one-half of all patients receiving lipid emulsion therapy.~~ Only about 1% of patients experience adverse reactions to lipid emulsion therapy.

3. ~~Late adverse reactions to lipid therapy include glucose in the urine, chills, malaise, leukocytosis, altered level of consciousness, elevated blood glucose levels, and fever.~~ These are signs and symptoms of sepsis, which can occur in any patient receiving a peripheral infusion.

6. ~~Lipids are extremely small and easily pass through I.V. tubing when administered as part of parenteral therapy.~~ Lipids are large fat globules that can clog I.V. tubing; all lipid emulsions that aren't given as part of the PPN solution but are piggybacked separately require the use of filters and controllers.

Page 200

Mind sprints

- Protein
- Carbohydrates
- Fat
- Electrolytes
- Micronutrients
- Vitamins
- Fluids

Strikeout

1. ~~Parenteral feeding therapy for children serves a dual purpose: maintaining the child's nutritional status and preventing inborn errors of metabolism.~~ Parenteral feedings in children help maintain the child's nutritional status and fuel growth; inborn errors of metabolism are inherited metabolic conditions that a child already has at birth.

4. ~~Hypoproteinemia can occur in infants receiving 20% lipid emulsions.~~ Thrombocytopenia (platelet deficiency) is associated with administering 20% lipid emulsions to infants.

■ Page 201

Power stretch

Sepsis: D, E
Clotted catheter: C, F
Catheter dislodgement: G
Cracked tubing: A
Pneumothorax: B, H

■ Page 202

Match point

1. D, 2. J, 3. E, 4. I, 5. C, 6. F, 7. A, 8. B, 9. H, 10. G

■ Page 203

Team up!

Hyperglycemia (high blood glucose): Anxiety, Coma, Confusion, Deliriousness, Fatigue, Restlessness, Weakness

Hypoglycemia (low blood glucose): Confusion, Irritability, Shaking, Sweating

Match point

1. D, 2. C, 3. A, 4. E, 5. F, 6. B

Notes

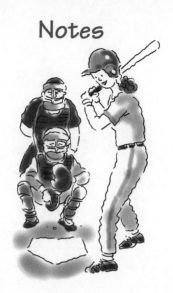

Notes

Notes

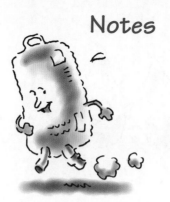

Notes

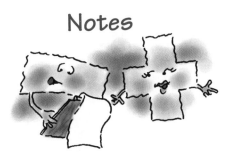

Notes

Notes

Notes

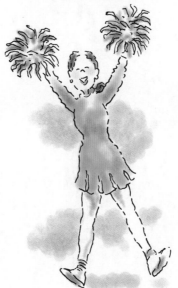

Notes

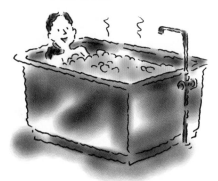

Notes

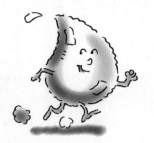